Shinjinbukan Shorin-ryu Karate-jutsu
神人武館小林流空手術

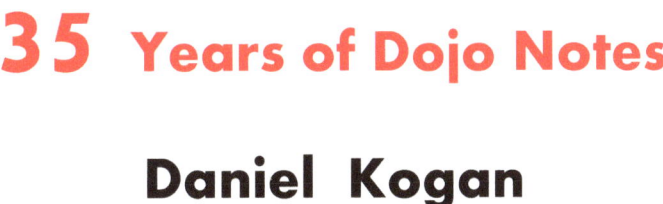

35 Years of Dojo Notes

Daniel Kogan

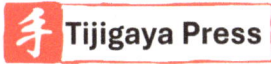
Tijigaya Press

Copyright 2024 © Daniel Kogan and Tijigaya Press

All rights reserved. No part of this work may be reproduced, republished, copied, or distributed without prior written permission from the author.

All content in this work is the sole property of the author. All images and illustrations, unless explicitly stated, are original work by the author.

Shinjinbukan Shorin-ryu Karate-jutsu: 35 Years of Dojo Notes
First Edition 2024
Text, photography, and layout by Daniel Kogan unless expressly noted otherwise.
Edited by Dr. Fara Nizamani

ISBN
979-8-9922768-0-0 (Paperback)

Contact information: info@tijigaya.com

Disclaimer
Training in the martial arts is inherently dangerous. The author and publisher of this book are not responsible in any way for any injury or trauma that may result from practicing or attempting to apply any of the techniques presented in this book. The content of this book is provided as a demonstration of how training is conducted at the Shinjinbukan and not as instructional material.

Front cover by the author: image of the Pine Lake Shibu Dojo 2023

Contents

	Page
Dedication	I
Acknowledgements	II

Preface 序章 *Introduction and reading guide*		1
Reigi 礼儀 *Dojo etiquette*		7
Yobi Undo 予備運動 *Preparatory exercises*		9
Hojo Undo 補助運動 *Supplementary exercises*		27
Kihon 基本 *Tsuki, Keri, Tenshin, hand and foot positions*		35
Tachi Gata 立ち型 *Stances*		45
Kushi Jike 腰突け *Hips*		51
Kamae 構え *Guards*		55
Kigu Undo 器具運動 *Equipment exercises*		59
Machiwara Undo マチワラ運動 *Standing Machiwara*		83
Sagi Machiwara サギマチワラ *Hanging Makiwara*		91
Yakusoku Kumite 約束組手 *Prearranged sparring*		99
Seiri Undo 整理運動 *Cool down*		105
Dojo No Naka 道場の中 *In the Dojo*		111
Kakemono 掛物 *Wall hangings, Dojo Kun, Nafuda*		117
Kata 型 *Forms*		121
Dani 段位 *Rank system*		125
Batsubun 跋文 *Epilogue*		135

Vocabulary ボキャブラリー	137

Dedication

To my teacher and my students, without whom I would be neither.

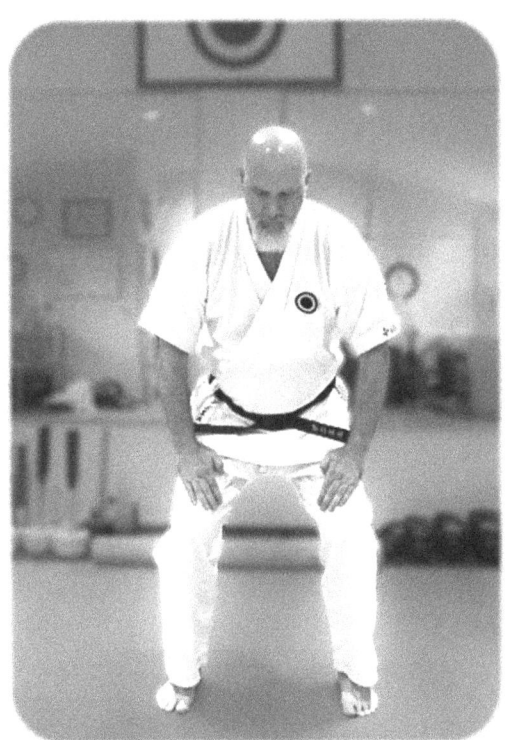

Acknowledgments

It goes without saying, and yet it seems odd to write this book about the Karate I have learned from my teacher and not expressly acknowledge all that Onaga Yoshimitsu sensei has done for me. Sensei took me in as a 20-year-old who knew nothing more than the trappings of Japanese sport Karate and, over the past 35 years, has taught, mentored, pushed, and motivated me to follow the path he has already walked, and to learn as much from his mistakes as from his accomplishments. None of the book, nor any of my Karate life, would have been possible if it were not for his countless hours spent and willingness to share with me that which took him a lifetime to learn and understand—I am forever in your debt. Thank you, sensei.

I also need to thank and acknowledge Dr. Timothy Black for the work reviewing early drafts of this manuscript and helping me decide what was valuable to include from a student's perspective. It was immeasurably valuable having a sounding board to help keep me on track as I worked through what to share in this manual. I could not have done this on my own, neither the book nor enduring following the path. Thank you, Tim.

Getting words on paper is a challenge but ultimately just effort. It's mostly in my head or on scraps of paper and handwritten notes. I've shared it all countless times during class, so it was just a matter of getting it done, but making the written work worthy of other people's time to read was another matter. I could not have completed this without the work and dedication of Dr. Fara Nizamani, who read, and reread many drafts providing assistance and guidance throughout the process. In spite of being warned upfront that Dr. Nizamani is ruthless with her red pen, it was not nearly as painful, at least for me, as I had first anticipated. Having someone who is not only skilled with the pen but has a grasp of the material was invaluable. Thank you, Fara.

I also want to thank Mr. Rick Dove, Mr. Vincent Liew, and Ms. Gabrielle Carson. Rick, Vincent, Gabrielle, along with Tim, represent my first generation of students. They took a bet on me over three decades ago and have stuck with me ever since. Thank you for pushing me when needed and supporting me when necessary. Most importantly, thank you for joining me on this journey of learning, growth, and understanding.

I would also like to acknowledge the help of Mr. Masaaki Sato with Japanese language translation and nuance that are always a challenge for anyone learning Okinawa Karate. Mr. Sato is a fellow student of Onaga sensei and good friend. Thank you, Masaaki san.

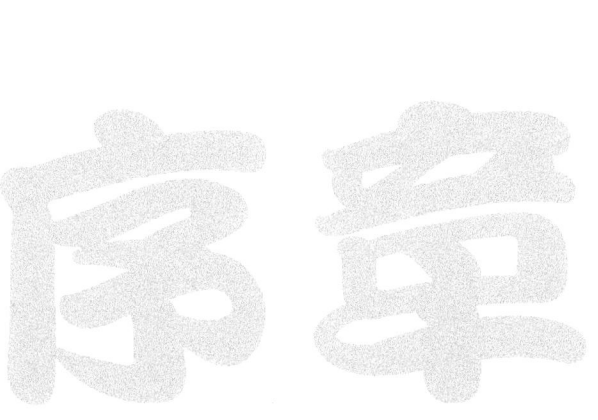
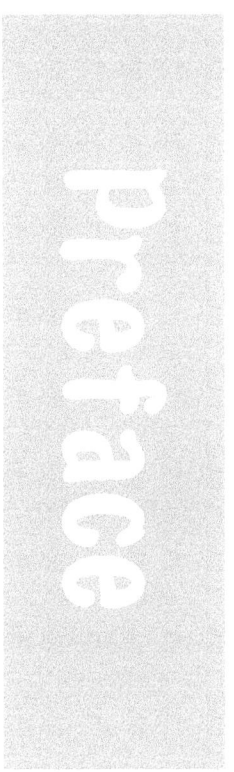

Preface

The idea for this student's manual came out of a recent project I did. I decided to make a poster with the Yobi Undo, in the order we use at our Dojo, with margin notes to help students recall what to think about while doing these exercises. I quickly realized I would need enough posters to wallpaper the average-sized Dojo if I wanted to document everything I wanted to convey. A small manual with the Yobi Undo seemed more reasonable and I thought each student could have their own and makes notes accordingly. That quickly grew to become this work with over 1000 images and transcription of my personal notes in the hope that it could help students along their journey. With that, let me clearly state what this book is not. It is not, and should not be seen as, a means to learn Karate. Karate, or Ti, cannot be learned from a book. This was repeatedly drilled into me when I lived in my teacher's Dojo in Okinawa and spent my free time scouring every used bookshop I could find on the island. This book, or any "Karate book," can only ever talk about Karate and should never pretend to teach or demonstrate real Karate.

So, what then is the purpose of this student manual? My hope is that it works as a reminder to students of the things they should be practicing. Many students simply just "follow along" during class. After all, it's the teacher's role to figure out what they should be working on. This "do as you're told approach" fails to understand one of the key concepts students need to grasp when stepping into the Dojo. Renshu (練習), or practice in Japanese, and Keiko (稽古), or training, are not the same thing, at least not as I was taught, and I have tried to teach my students this key difference.

Renshu is what the student does. They practice what they are taught. Keiko is what the teacher does in that they "train" the student. In other words, you receive training, then you practice what you've learned.

Most students get stuck when told to practice on their own. Hopefully this student manual will be of some help when students have time to practice. When the teacher is teaching, students won't need this book; they should just do as they are instructed. But far too often, if the teacher is not handing out tasks and counting, students will pause. This was never the case at the Onaga Dojo. In fact, students are often in the Dojo practicing the most recent thing they learned, be that 10 minutes ago or 2 nights ago. Being able to practice on one's own is important, but it can be difficult.

I have spent years taking notes after class and getting them reviewed by my teacher. I have also spent nearly as much time encouraging my students to take notes. At the end of the day, learning Karate is an individual pursuit, much like a traveler taking notes and journalling along their travels, I think students should record their journey along *the way* (道), since these notes are what will allow the student to revisit, relive, and reexamine where they've been and what they've learned along the way.

During class, I often heard sensei remind me that the teacher's job is to fix what a student is doing wrong, to show the student the path the teacher has taken so they can follow, and to offer up a menu of ideas from which they can pick. Since no two students are the same, they may follow the same path but focus on different things along the way.

It is in the spirit of presenting a menu of ideas that this student's manual is provided. It is not an exhaustive list of ideas or exercises. It is not a resource a student should reach for when trying to learn a new concept or technique. Rather, it is a memory crutch for when a student is looking to recall some exercise or concept in order to practice what they've been taught. It is hoped that this collection of images with brief explanations might also be the nudge some students need to start documenting their own journey in the Dojo.

I have known very few serious Karateka who don't closely guard their countless volumes of notebooks. I've seen fellow Karateka whose notebooks are masterpieces of both artistic detail, and deep knowledge. At first I found it difficult to write down all the detail I was receiving. There was just too much and it was often hard to know where to start. I even ended up developing my own form of shorthand in order to be able to draw and scribble Karate concepts quickly and consistently because I knew I would need to make sense of them years later.

It's been close to forty years of note taking with pen and paper. Although most of my note taking is still primarily done with paper and pen, technology has allowed me to document things in a much different way. In the early 1990s, I made a point of filming my Kata, just for my own reference, and as a way to augment the volumes of notes I had taken in my time living in the Onaga Karate Dojo. But without narration, the videos lack the detail I was able to capture on the page, and yet, without the video, I was always concerned that I might miss something or misremember — so I did both, detailed handwritten notes as well as videos.

I have repeated documenting my Kata every 10 years or so as I have learned more and better understood what I should have been doing in the first place. That has been my journey and the method I chose for myself. I push my students to take notes because that has been my chosen path and, as mentioned, one job a teacher has is to show students the path the teacher has taken, so the students can follow it if they choose.

I realized at an early age that the amount of content and knowledge imparted by Onaga sensei was too much and came at me too fast to digest in real time, and sensei realized it as well. He would often instruct me to remember what I was hearing or seeing because I would need to be able to recall it later when I might be more prepared to better understand it. Training was often capturing what at the time seemed like disjointed ideas and concepts, knowing that they were in fact connected, but I just wasn't quite able to see how yet. And so, not trusting it to memory alone, I took notes. I don't think I'm unique in this regard. Every Karateka, to a one, who in my opinion has been able to learn the deep meaning of what they've been taught, has piles of notebooks, scrap papers, and, yes, videos.

Staring at a blank page can be overwhelming, whereas adding one's own notes, impressions, thoughts, memories, and experiences to the pages of this student's manual will hopefully be easier than starting anew. I have intentionally provided space on the pages and included a few blank pages, in the hope that students use it like a workbook and not a bookshelf ornament.

As mentioned, this manual is not intended to teach Karate. It is a reference manual for students to get a glimpse of how things are done in my Dojo. It's important to note that there is no single "right way" to do things. There are certainly better and worse ways, there are familiar or novel ways, there is no shortage of examples of wrong ways, but there is no such thing as "the right way." Body-type is often a defining or limiting factor. Each student is on their own journey of understanding, and the milestones they've reached will have a huge impact on what can and should be expected from them. In the same Dojo, training in front of their teacher, two students may be doing things notably differently and yet neither gets corrected, as both could in fact be correct for where they are at in their individual journeys.

Teaching and learning Karate is a very personal journey. The goal of a teacher should not be to transmit or to produce a standardized curriculum that others would recognize as a "style" but rather to provide the tools and techniques that each individual student both needs and can apply when their life is on the line. For the student, training and learning should not be about preserving, but rather finding ways to be able to apply the knowledge. With that in mind, what a teacher gives each student may differ. This can sometimes be a complicated and frustrating aspect of training in a traditional Dojo. What you are doing may not look like what the person next to you is doing, and I've heard many foreigners complain about how teachers keep changing things, as if this was being done to them to deliberately keep them off balance and ensure they never really *get it*. It is mostly foreigners, primarily Westerners, because they have both the burden and the benefit of being able to question what is taught to them. This is typically not the case with junior ranks of Japanese or Okinawan students who usually have more deference to authority and typically accept what is taught with little or no question.

The reason students often feel that teachers keep moving the goal posts is because they lack the perspective the teacher has to see the different needs across individuals or across time. As students improve, a more difficult or subtly-nuanced version of an idea or technique is introduced to take advantage of the newly-acquired skill. Or alternatively, after significant effort has been applied trying to perfect and polish something to no avail, the teacher might decide to modify the technique to make it more practical, rather than having the technique remain simply theoretical and unattainable for that particular student.

I will leave the responsibility for the teaching and the training to each student's direct instructor, and hope to provide some assistance in preparing the student for their own practice with this notebook to help jumpstart what will, hopefully, become a lifetime of note taking.

Reading Notes

This student manual is not intended to be a language course. The use of Japanese is primarily to assist with context and meaning and doesn't pretend to try to teach students the Japanese language in any kind of meaningful way. Rather, it is there to assist in conveying the ideas presented.

As such, the romanization of Japanese terms is not done in an academically rigorous way, so there are times when long vowel sounds are missed or short or double consonants are left out. The spelling used is the English language approximation of the Japanese or Okinawan as most commonly found in Dojo in North America. This is for no other reason than to help students match what they might see during class on the whiteboard or online, and not to suggest that these are the "correct" terms, but rather the common ones.

Language does matter, and when it does there is an attempt throughout the manual to call it out, either by showing the Japanese ideogram (Kanji) or by other means, but keep in mind that this manual is not a language course.

Reading K and G

Through out the book you will notice that often the letters K and G appear to be interchangeable. For example, the Kanji for Kata 型 is read "Kata" when it is a single word, but "Gata" when it is in phrase or compound word. "Keri" and "Geri", and "Kamae" and "Gamae" are other common examples of this hard consonant sound being softened when found in the middle of a compound word.

Capitalization

Japanese words written in English, or what is referred to as "Romaji" in Japanese, are capitalized throughout this text. This is standard practice when using Japanese words in English writing. Exceptions were made for a few titles like "sensei" and "san" which for some reason seem awkward when capitalized and as a result have intentionally been written with lower case letters.

Pluralization

Japanese words used in English are usually not pluralized. This can sometimes result in the English sentences appearing malformed, but this is usually due to a lack of context rather than a grammar issue. For example, Yobi Undo and Seiri Undo are used as singular nouns, as each is thought of as a single set, while Hojo Undo and Kigu Undo are viewed as categories of exercises and tend to be plural, even though that is sometimes not obvious in English.

Reading Notes

Understanding the symbols used

In general, both the photographs and symbols should be able to stand alone with little to no explanation. As mentioned previously, the intent is not to teach but to help students remember and focus on specific aspects of their training. As the saying goes, "a picture is worth a thousand words." Most of the images in this manual are provided for students to review and, hopefully, add their own margin notes where needed, with little more than a few pointers from me.

That said, there has been an attempt made to standardize the following uses of symbols overlayed on the photographs.

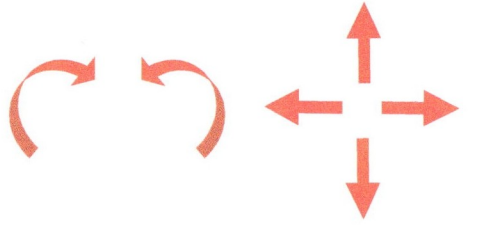

The use of arrows, straight, curved, or angled, all indicate direction. Either the movement of a technique, the direction where pressure or focus is applied, or where the eyes should be looking.

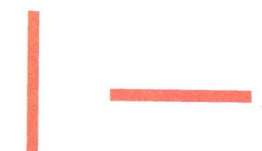

Solid lines are used to indicate a static position or alignment.

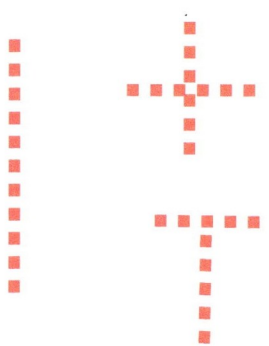

Dashes indicate a way to measure or check one's position.

The red square or rectangle shows where a surface area makes contact.

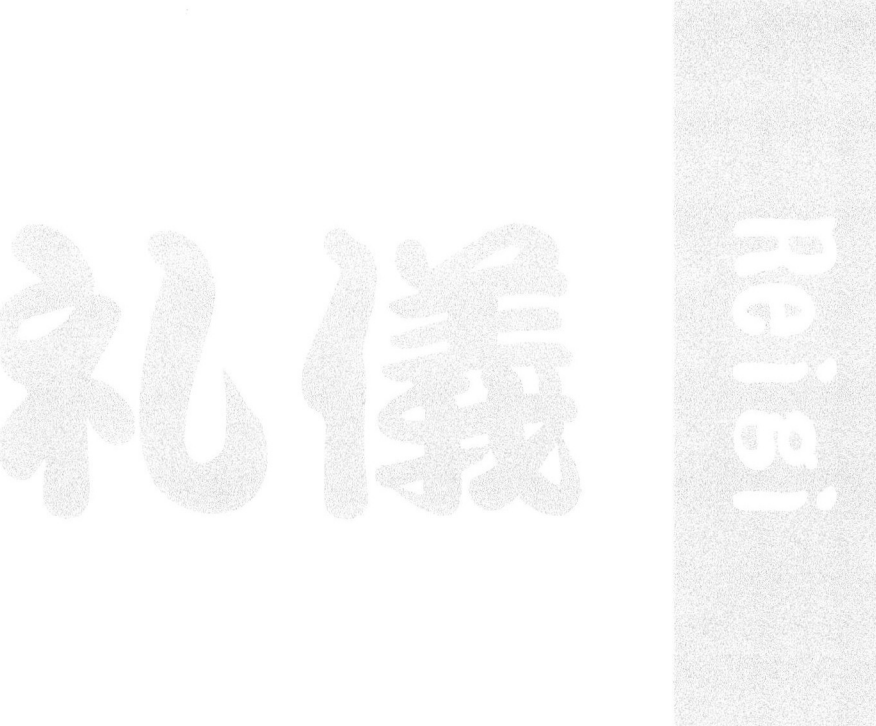

When entering the Dojo, be it a room at the local school or community center, an outdoor training area, or a dedicated space, bow before you enter. If your sensei is already present, wait to be acknowledged and given permission to enter.

Bowing is both a sign of respect and a deliberate expression of gratitude. During class, students rarely speak. When shown a technique, or when provided with an explanation or an example, rather than saying "thank you," a simple and slow bow expresses the student's feelings. Bowing is done in direct response to an action or request, or out of the student's own initiative to express themselves.

Bowing is typically done in the direction of someone, with the exception of bowing towards Shomen (front of the Dojo) to close class; otherwise, a student will usually turn to face the instructor to thank them with a bow. When finishing Kata, you might turn to the instructor at the end and bow to acknowledge the teaching. Bowing is not part of the Kata; we do not start or finish a Kata with a bow. This is often confusing for students because they see their seniors bowing before and after Kata, but they are missing the context. Often a student will bow when receiving an instruction, for example, "Please perform Naihanchi Kata" and then again at the end of the Kata to express their appreciation for the lessons taught.

Reigi

礼儀

Upon entering the Dojo to begin training, kneel in Seiza (正座) position prior to stepping on the Dojo floor, then bow and request permission to enter by saying, "Onegaishimasu."

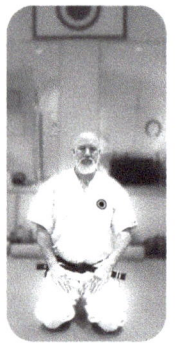 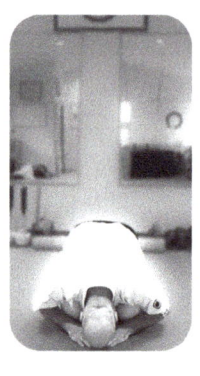 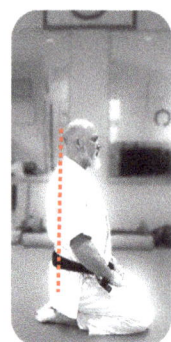 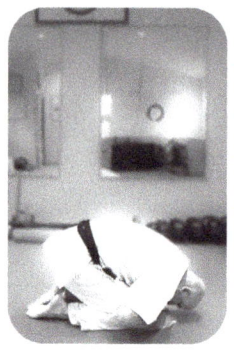

If class has started, wait for an opportunity to request permission to enter; otherwise just call out "Onegaishimasu" and wait for the teacher to acknowledge you and grant permission to enter.

The standard form of bowing is done at two levels, depending on the intent. This is used in daily life in Japan and is not unique to the Dojo.

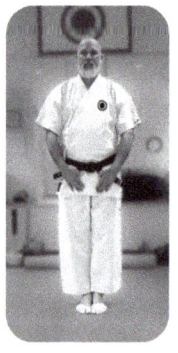 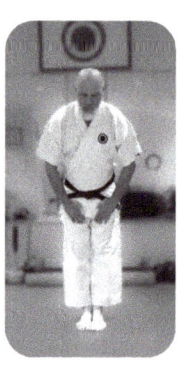 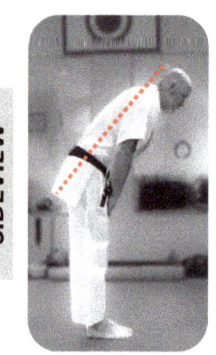 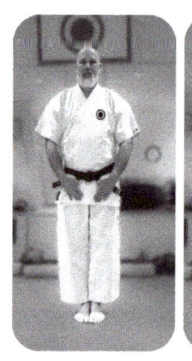 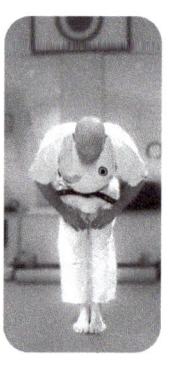 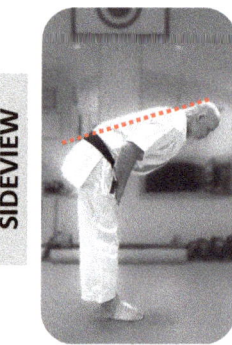

Bending the knees is a very old form of showing respect and not common in modern Dojo.

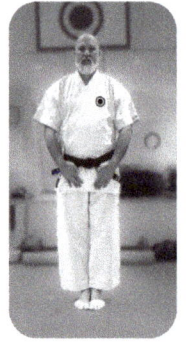 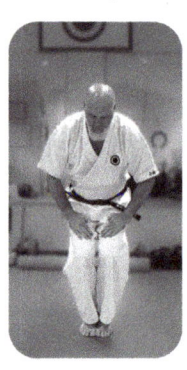 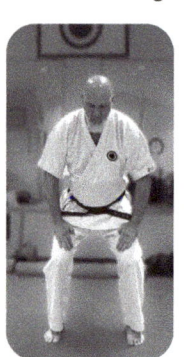 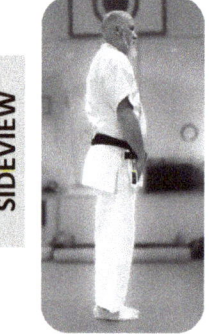 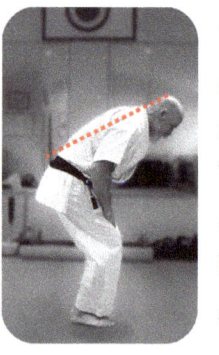

This form of bowing is done both with the feet together or apart. The feet together is considered the more humble of the two and akin to the deep bow common in Japanese culture today.

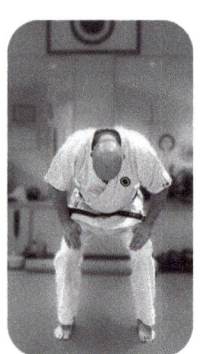

Typically, the head does not drop unless in a very intentional gesture to express submissiveness or absolute trust.

Yobi Undo (予備運動), or preparatory exercises, in some Dojo is referred to as Junbi Undo (準備運動) but the difference, although subtle, is important. Yobi Undo is intended to have a direct, 1-to-1 connection between each exercise and a specific movement or concept in Karate and, hence, is done in "preparation" for Karate. Yobi Undo should be seen as reinforcing the Karate techniques, whereas Junbi Undo is a focus on stretching and limbering up; in other words, a warmup. Students are free to find ways to warm up that suit their specific needs, but the Yobi Undo is done in a prescribed order and count. Each set is counted out in sets of eight.

Typically each set in the Yobi Undo is done twice (2x8) for every exercise. The Yobi Undo is done before every class or individual practice, usually on one's own. After entering the Dojo, a student will find a place on the Dojo floor to complete the Yobi Undo, since there is no need, or expectation, for class to be "formally" started. Students need to "prepare" for class, and the teacher will often wait until students have completed the preparatory exercises before starting class. If students complete the Yobi Undo, it is their responsibility to begin individual practice until class starts. Junior students who haven't committed the Yobi Undo series to memory will follow their sempai (先輩, senior). Yobi Undo is the first thing students need to commit to memory.

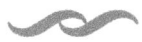

予備運動 Yobi Undō

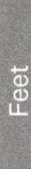

Feet

Big toe moves independently from the other toes.

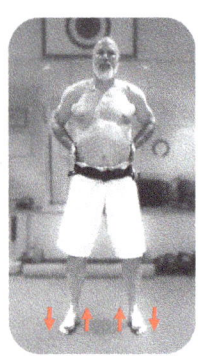 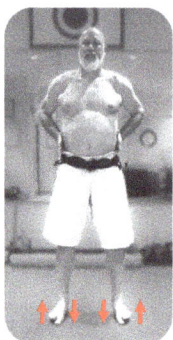 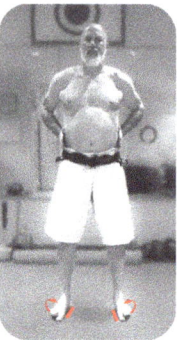 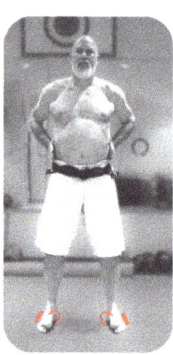 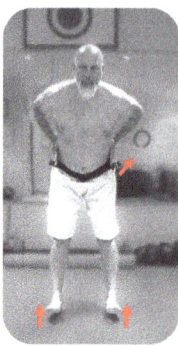 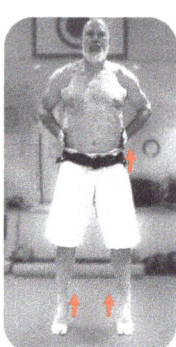

SIDEVIEW

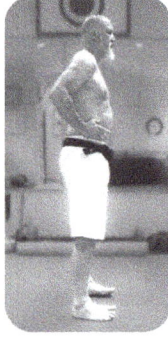 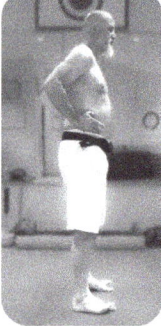 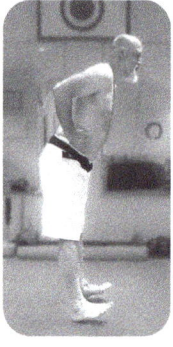

When rocking back on the heels, the hips push back.

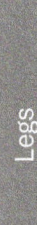

Legs

Roll the extended leg outwards.

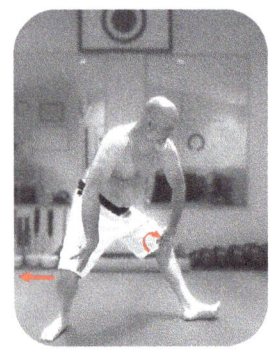 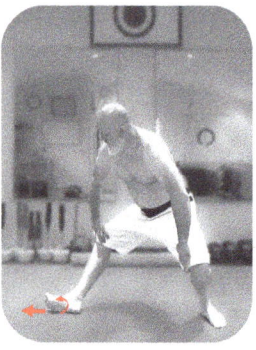 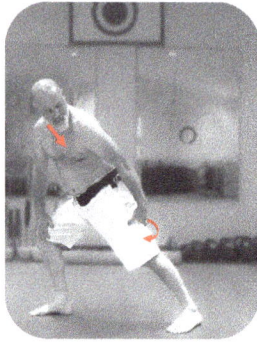

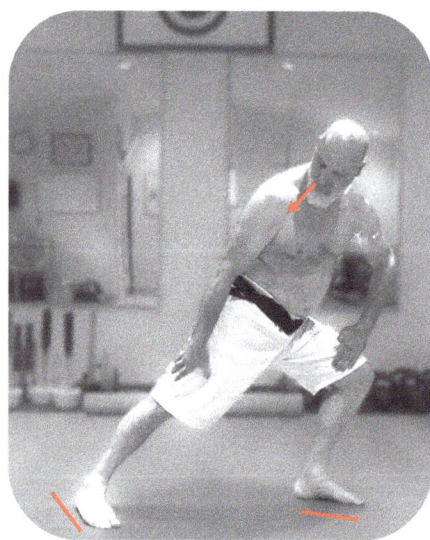

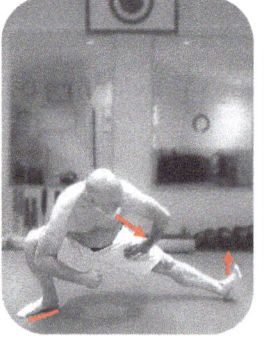 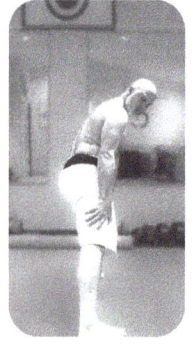

SIDEVIEW

Look towards the extended leg.

予備運動　　　Yobi Undō

Pushing the knees against the hands. Grip the patella and relax before changing direction.

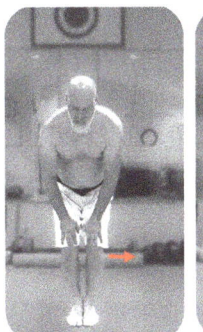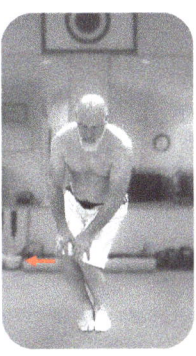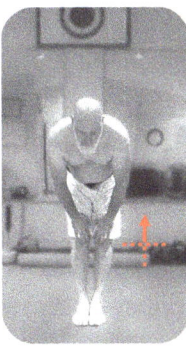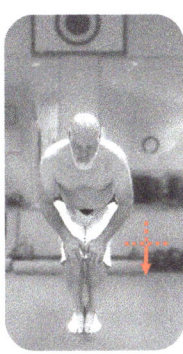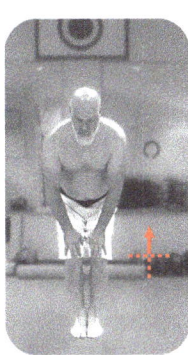

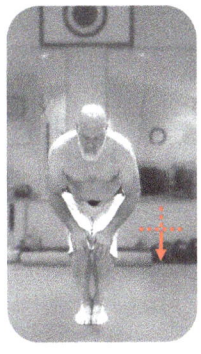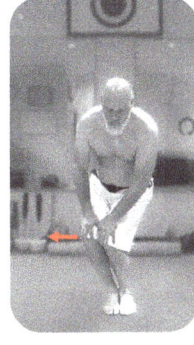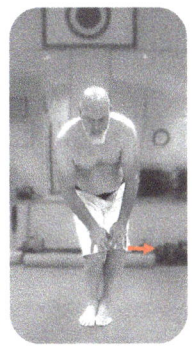

Knee rotations

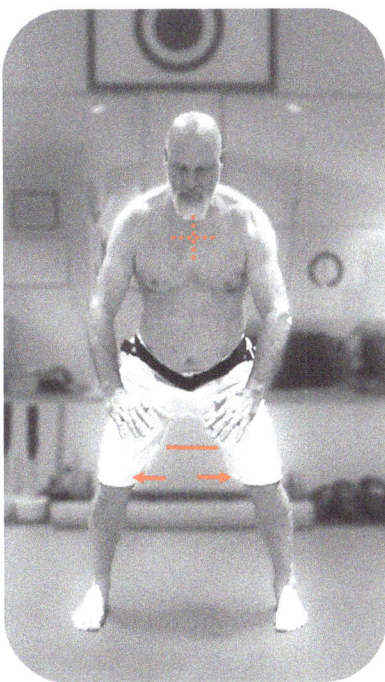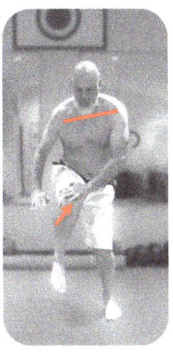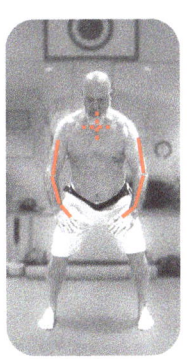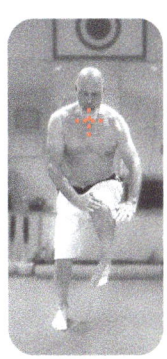

Strike the hand with the knee across the body. Try not to move your arms and shoulders.

Knees up

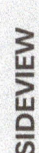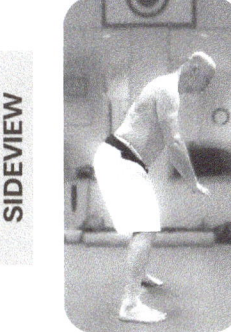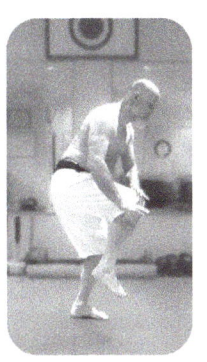

SIDEVIEW

予備運動　　　　　　　　　　　　　　　　　　Yobi Undō

Focus on the hip moving directly forward, to sides and back, with the leg straight. Once both sides are completed, repeat as a single circular movement forward and backwards.

Hips

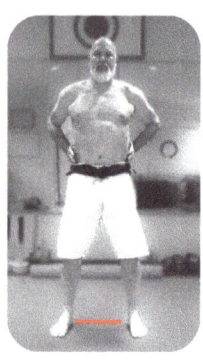 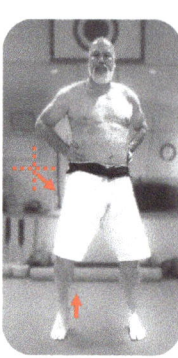 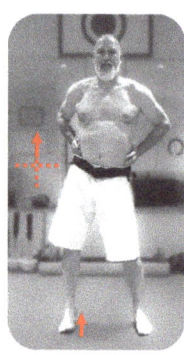 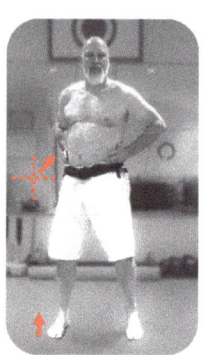

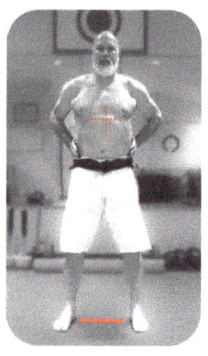 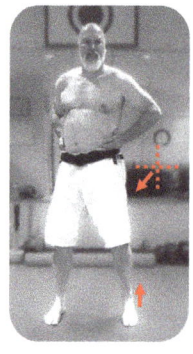 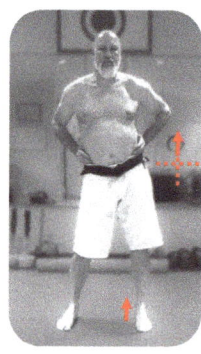 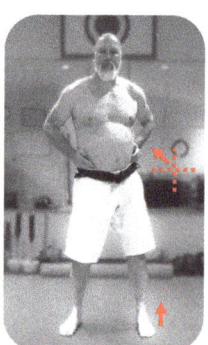

SIDEVIEW

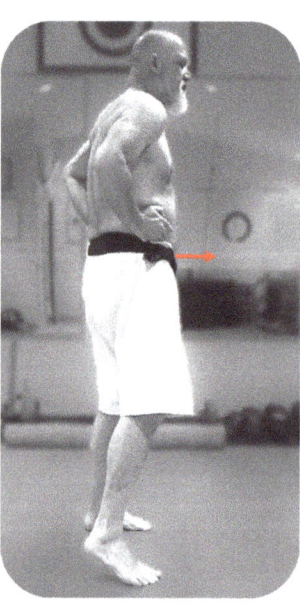 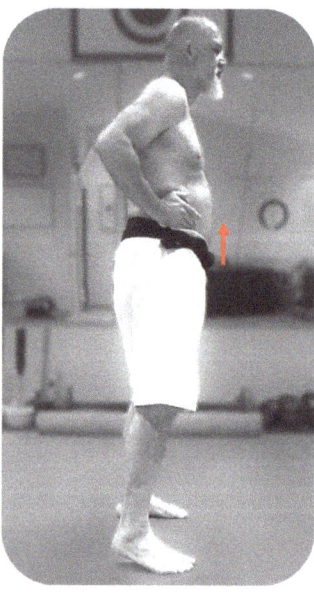 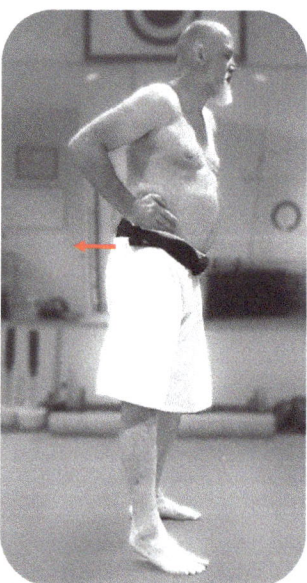

予備運動　　　　　　　　　　　　Yobi Undō

Leg raises

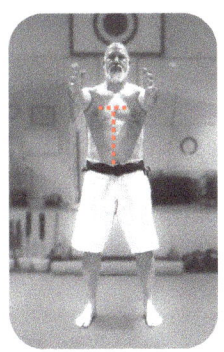 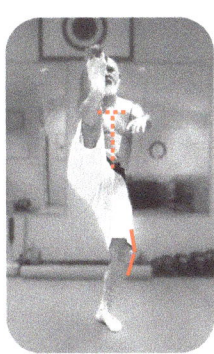 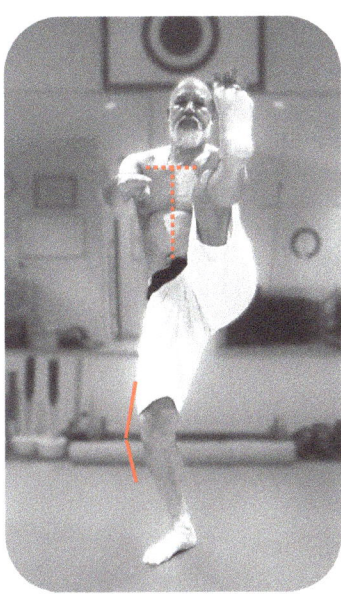

On all leg raises and circles, lower the leg as slowly and as controlled as possible.

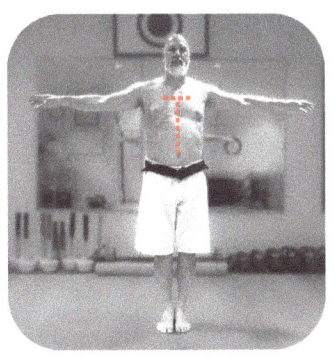 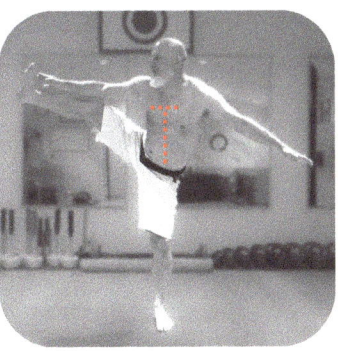 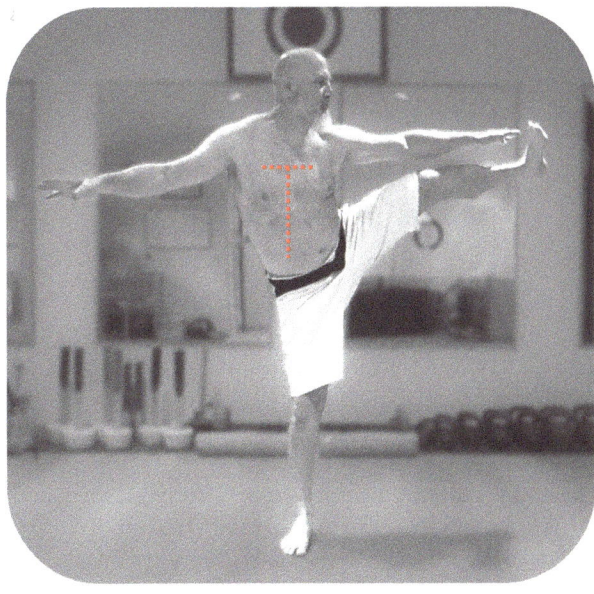

予備運動 Yobi Undō

Focus on opening the hip during the rotation.

Outward circles

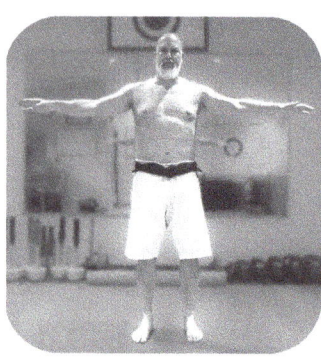 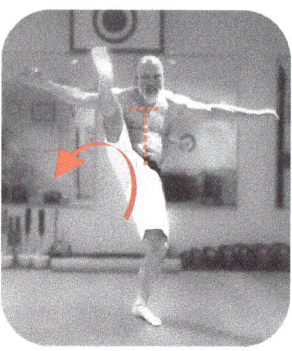 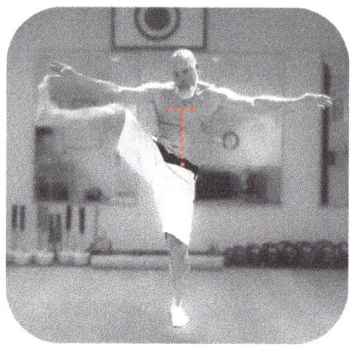 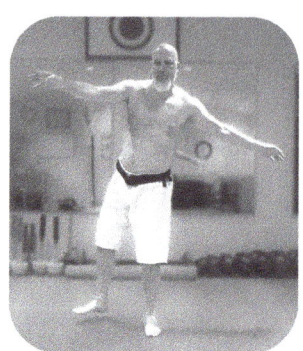

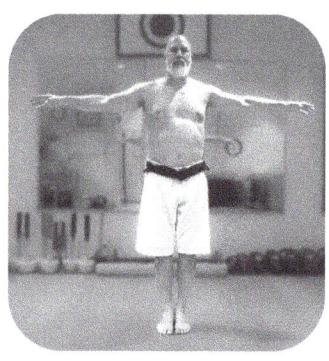 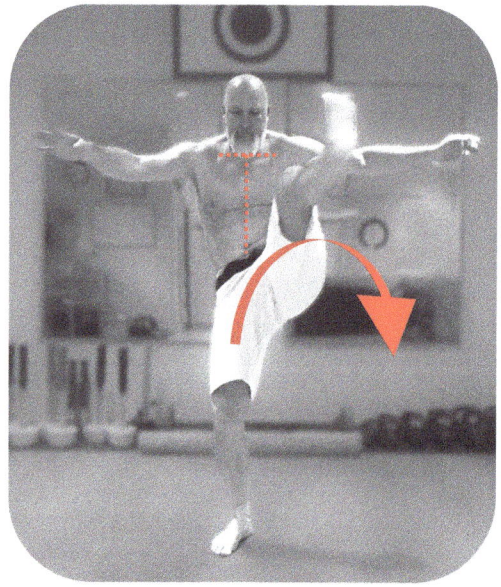

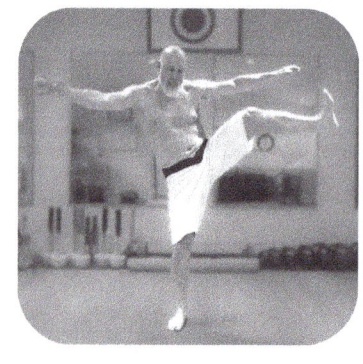 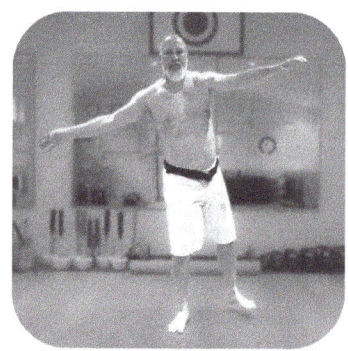

予備運動 — Yobi Undō

Start the rotation from the outside, not the front.

Inward circles

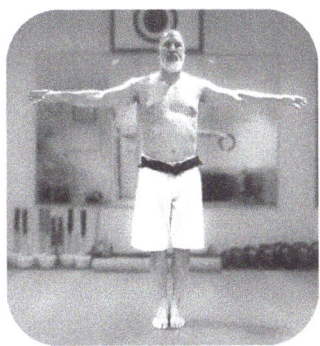
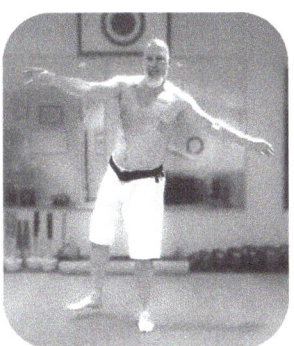
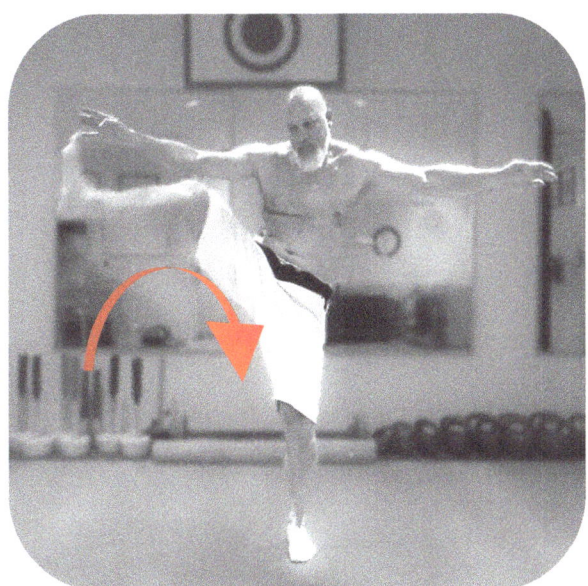
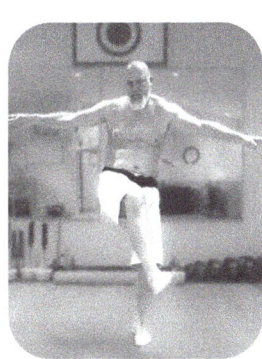
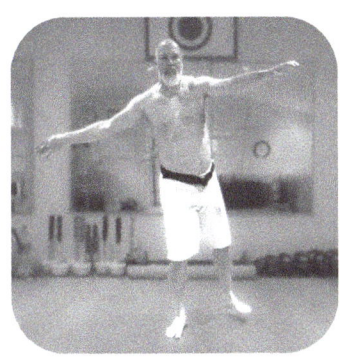
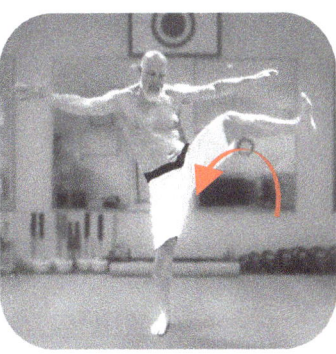
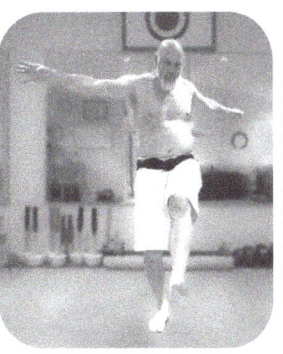
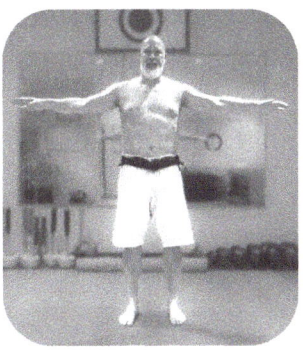

予備運動　Yobi Undō

Each hand position corresponds to a specific focus point on the feet as you squat down.

Squats

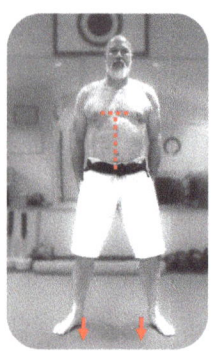 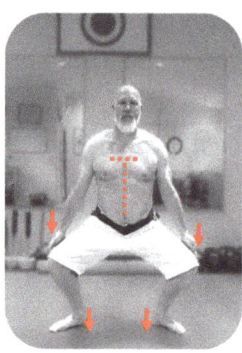 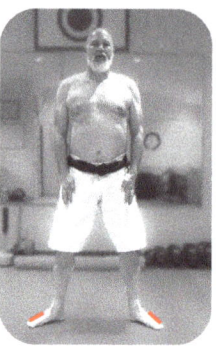 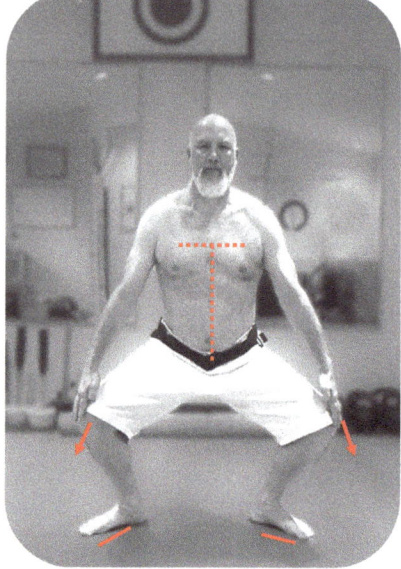

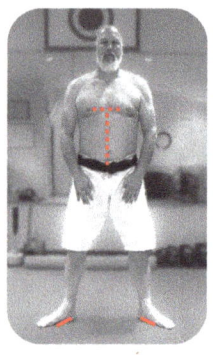 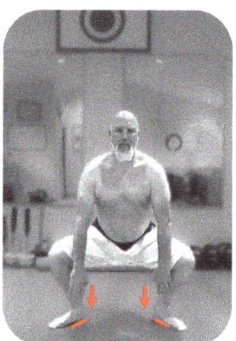

SIDEVIEW

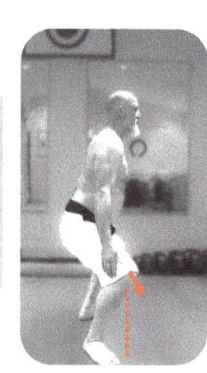 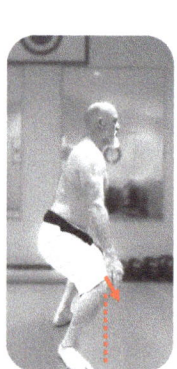 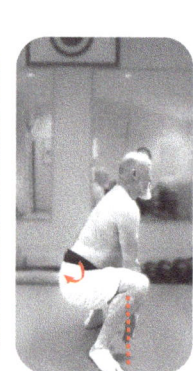

予備運動　　　　　　　　　　　　　　　Yobi Undō

Push the shoulder forward, in, and down.

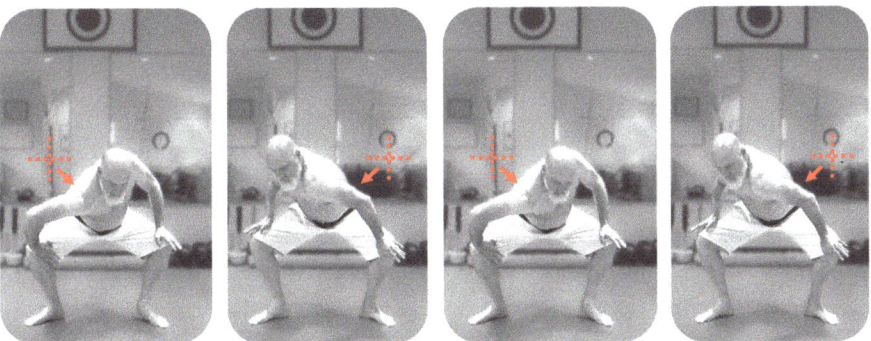

Roll onto the heels shifting the weight.

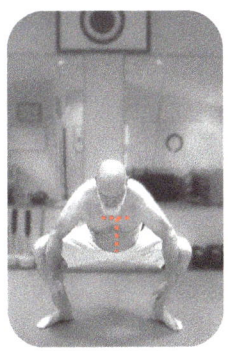 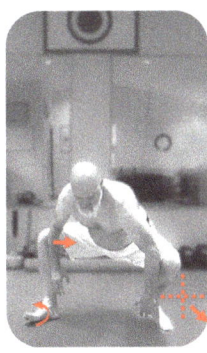 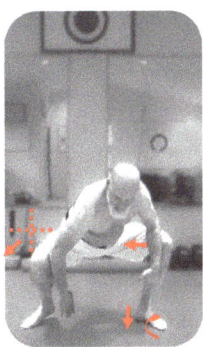 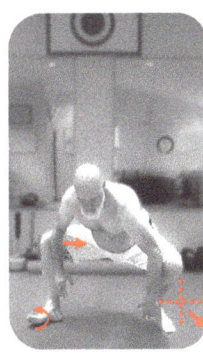 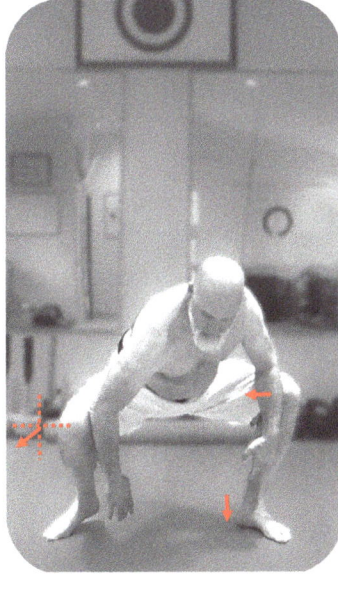

予備運動   Yobi Undō

Twist the body from the hips to the shoulders, reaching across to the opposite side, and look up at the hand.

Torso twists

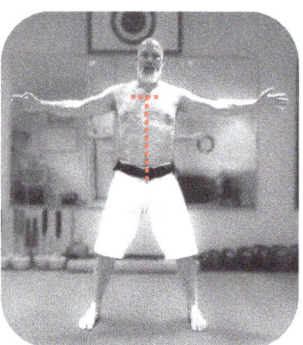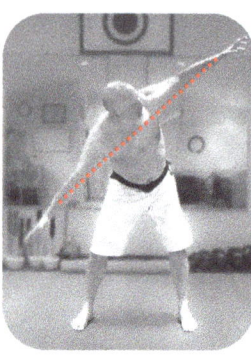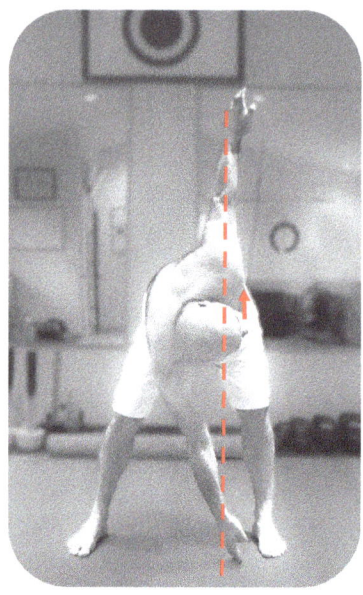

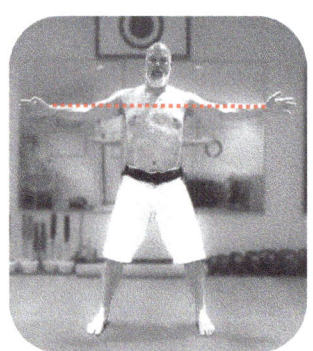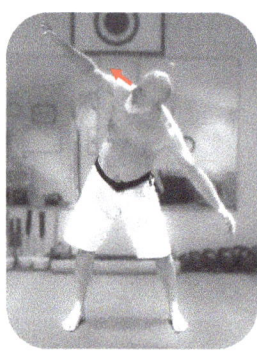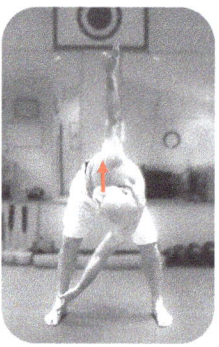

Expand the chest as you reach back.

SIDEVIEW

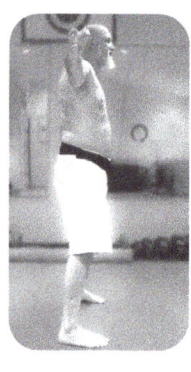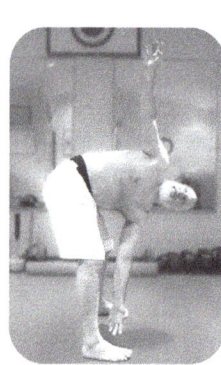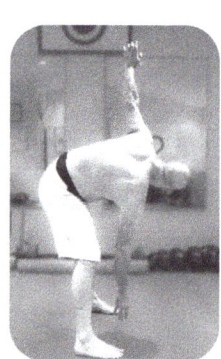

予備運動　　　　　　　　　　　　　Yobi Undō

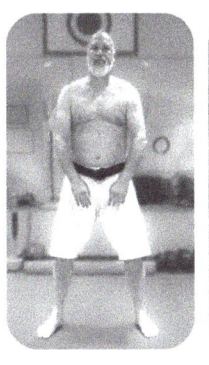 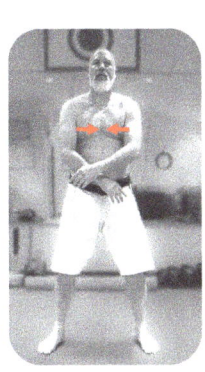 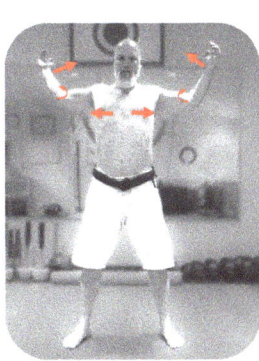 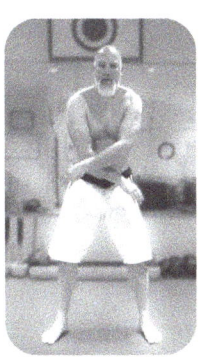 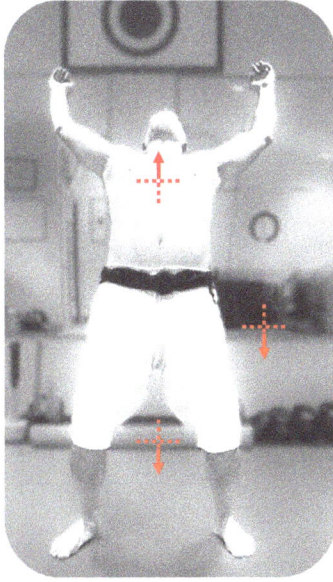

Chest

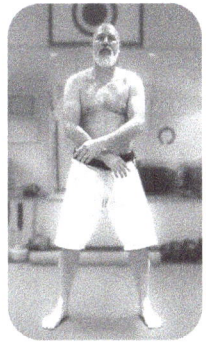 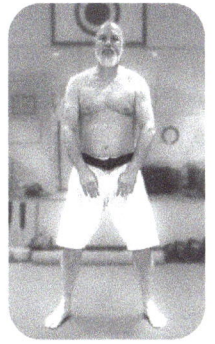

SIDEVIEW

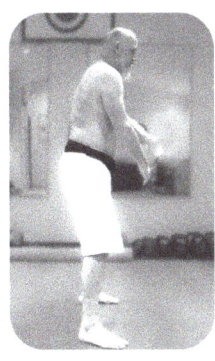 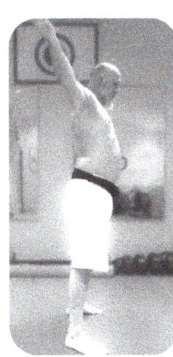 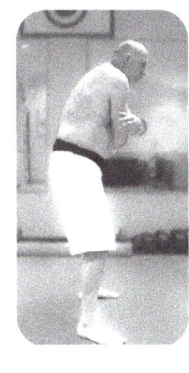 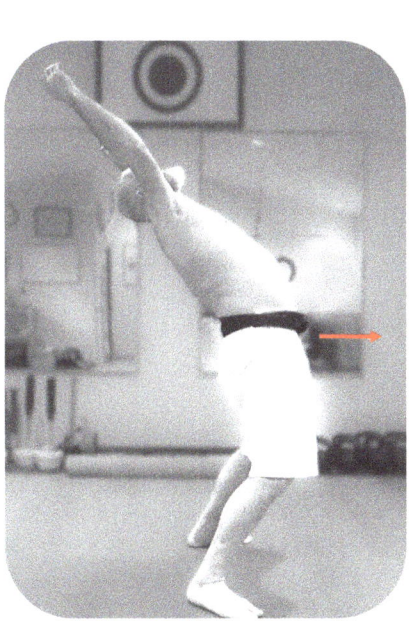

Push the hips forward and look at the wall behind you.

予備運動 Yobi Undō

Back tilt

Arms and legs slightly flexed. Push the hips forward and look at the wall behind you.

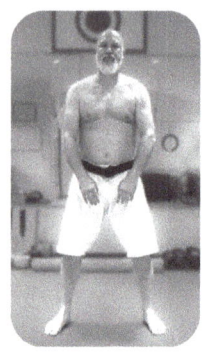
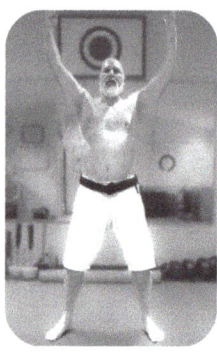
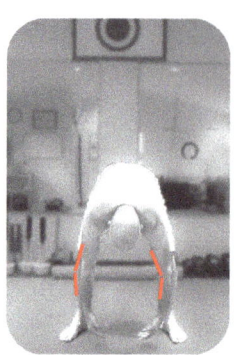
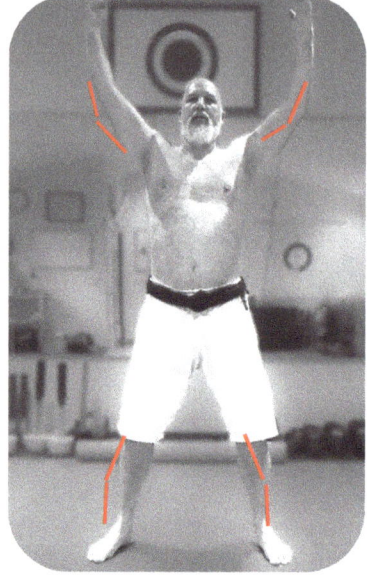
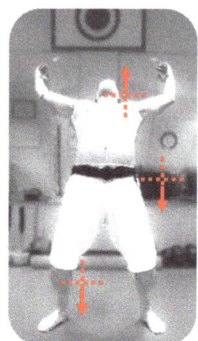

SIDEVIEW

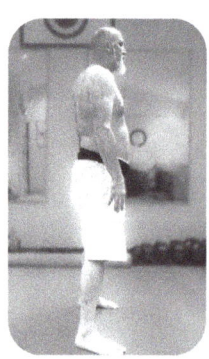
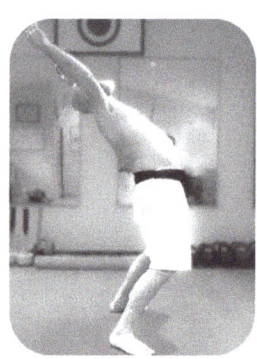
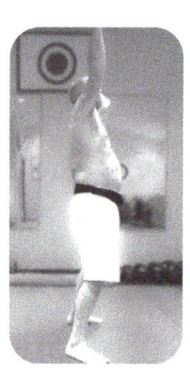
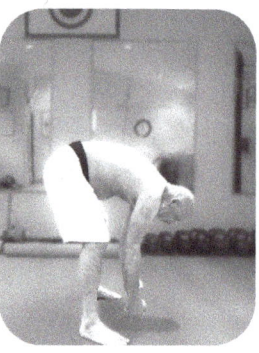

予備運動 Yobi Undō

Pull the arms back down by contracting the lats, not just lowering the hand.

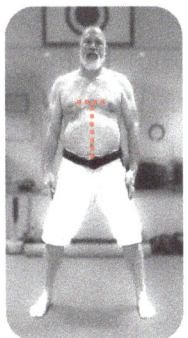
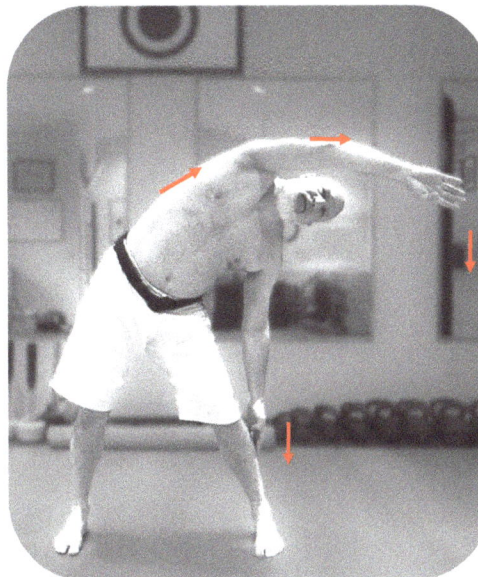
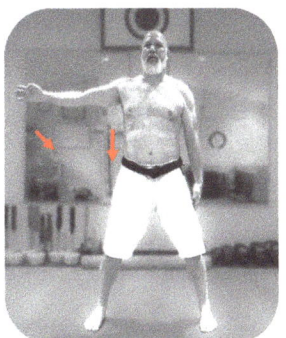

Lateral tilt

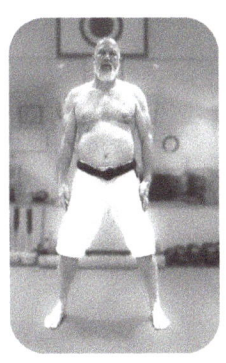
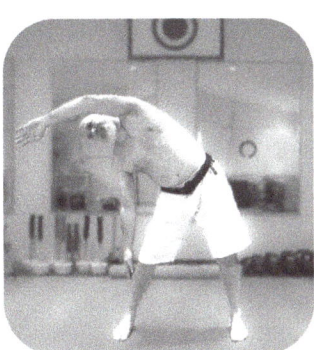
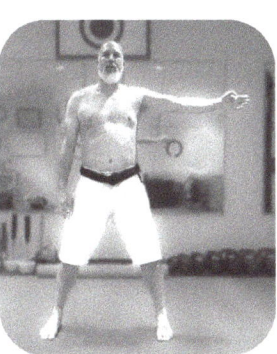
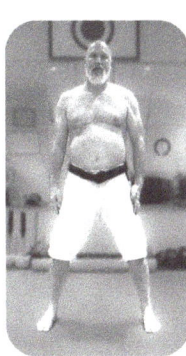

予備運動 — Yobi Undō

Torso rotations

Arms and legs slightly flexed.

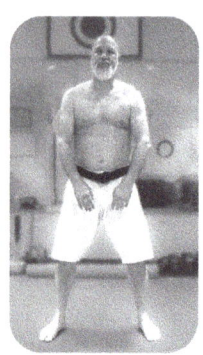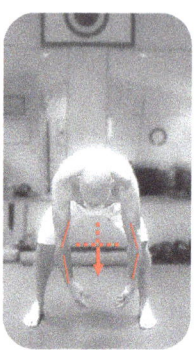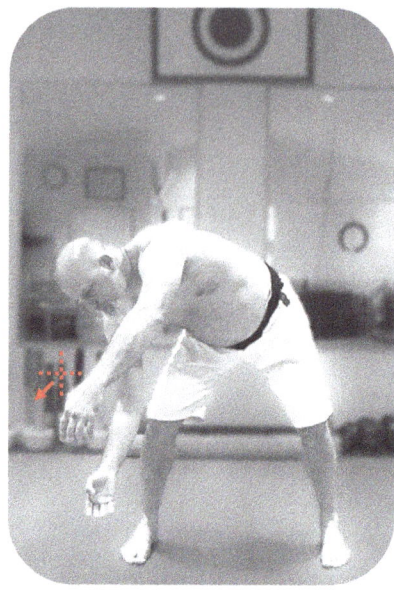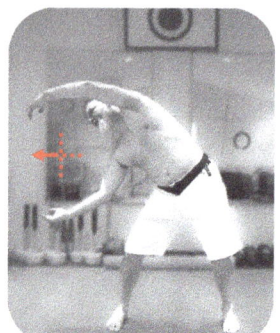

Smooth, full circle while paying attention to each of the 8 directions.

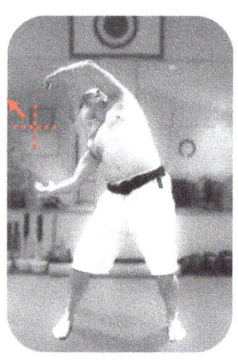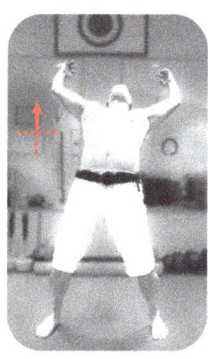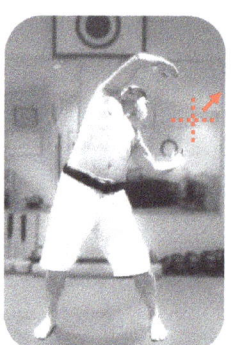

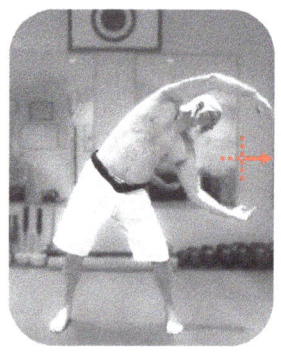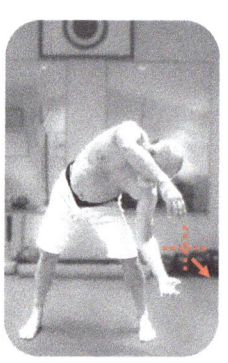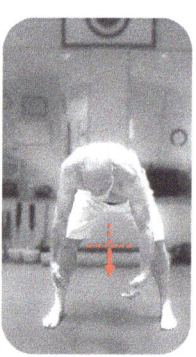

予備運動 Yobi Undō

Rotate the arms from the lats and the hands (thumbs) simultaneously.

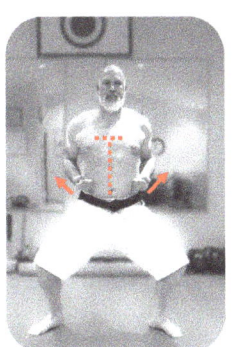 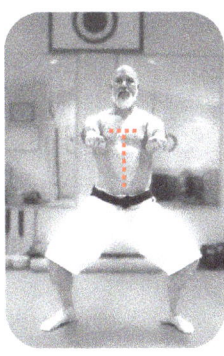 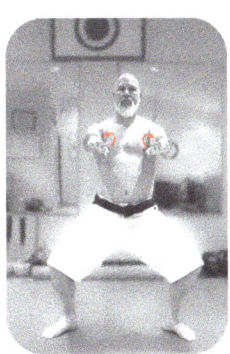 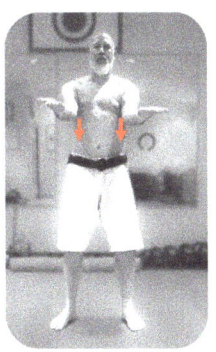 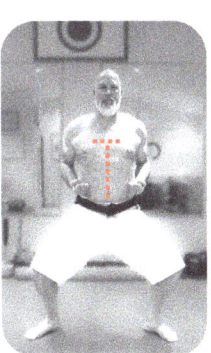

Arms

The arms follow the timing of the hips.

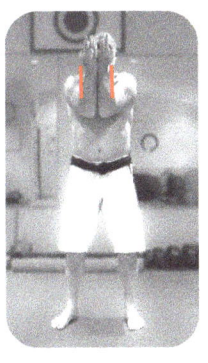 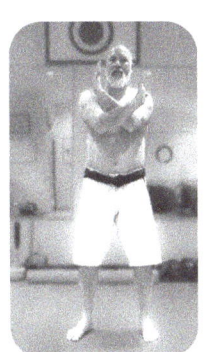 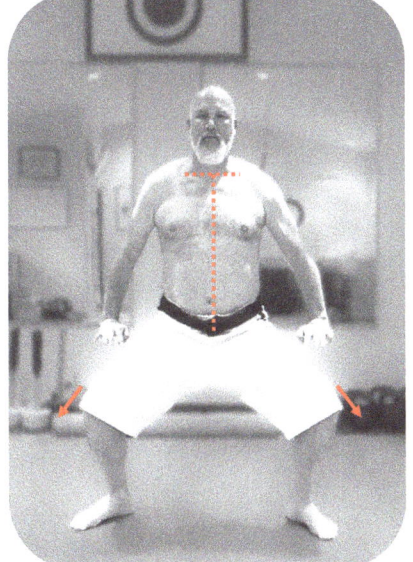 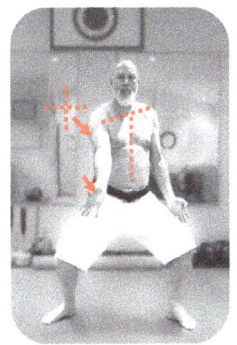

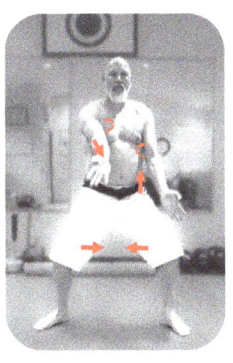 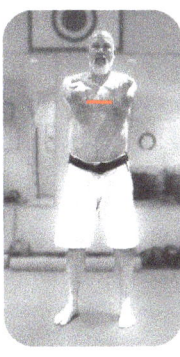 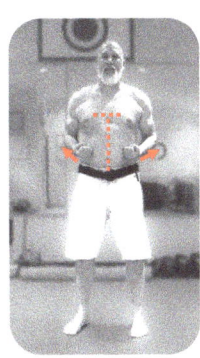 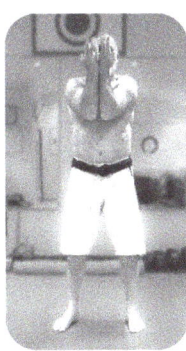

予備運動　　　　Yobi Undō

Hands

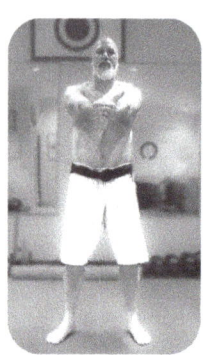 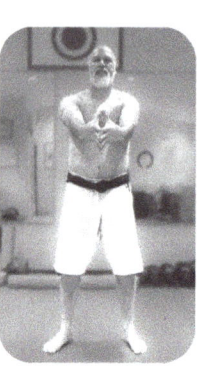 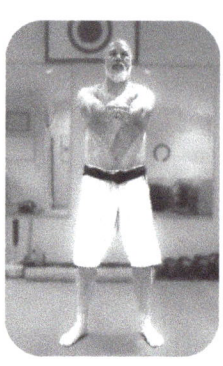 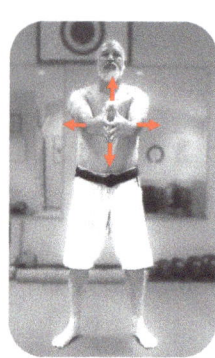

Thumbs and fingers are spread out as much as possible when the hands are in front of the chest.

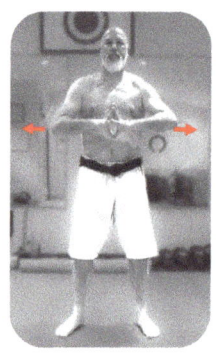 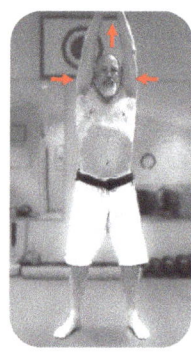

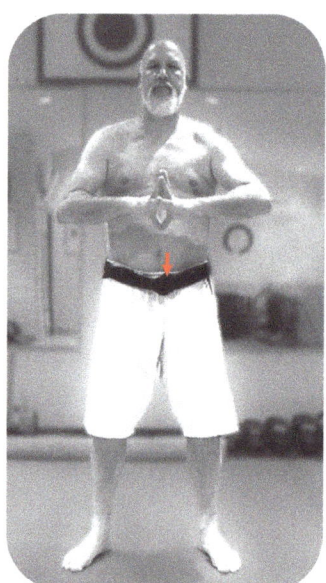

Biceps by the ears when the arms are pointing up.

予備運動　Yobi Undō

Keep your eyes level as you turn.

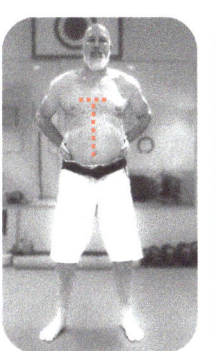 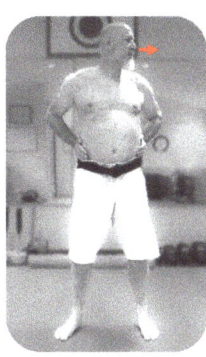 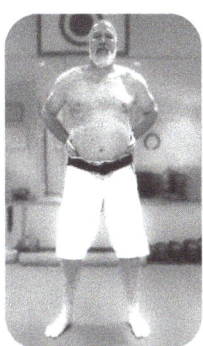 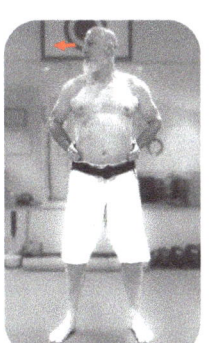 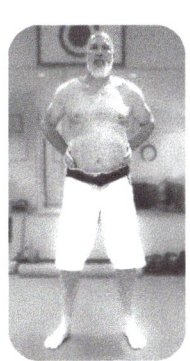

Neck

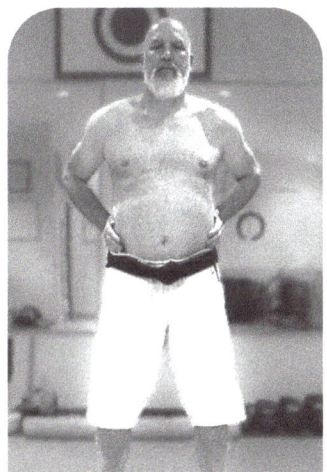 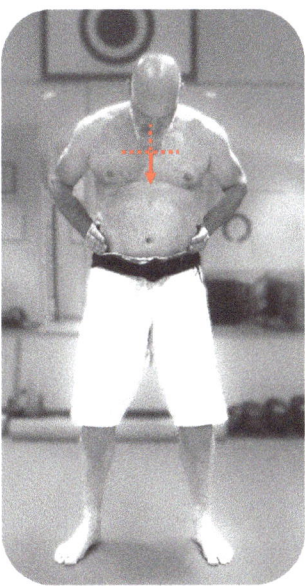 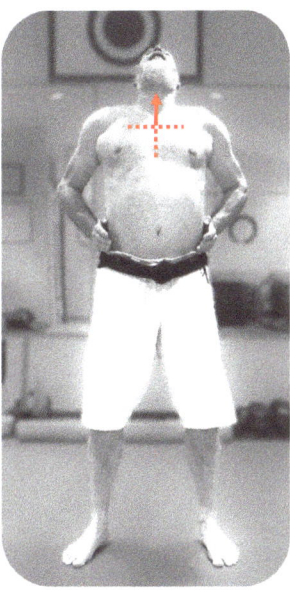 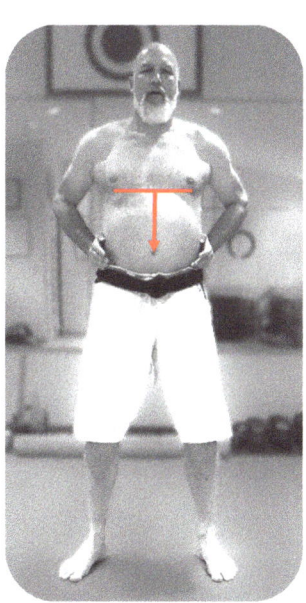

        Exhale.   Inhale.   Forced exhalation.

25

Yobi Undō

予備運動

Neck

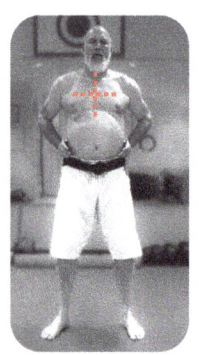 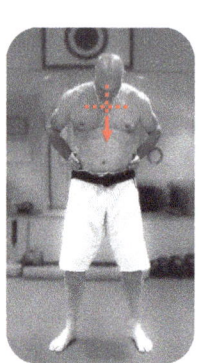 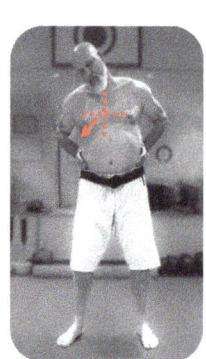 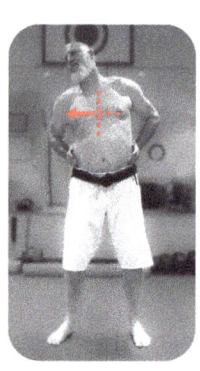 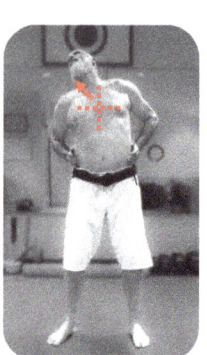

Eyes lead the movement of the head.

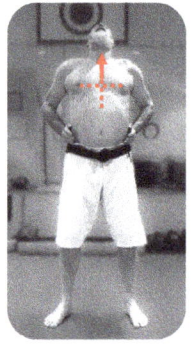 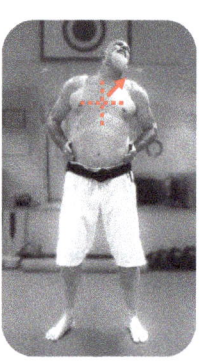 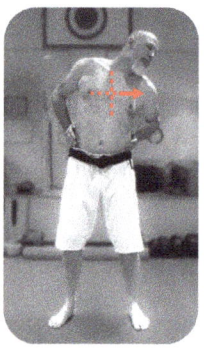 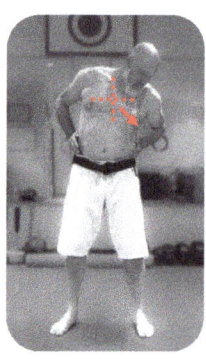 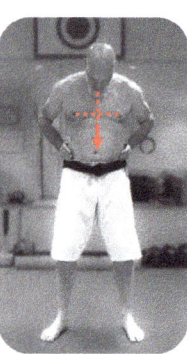

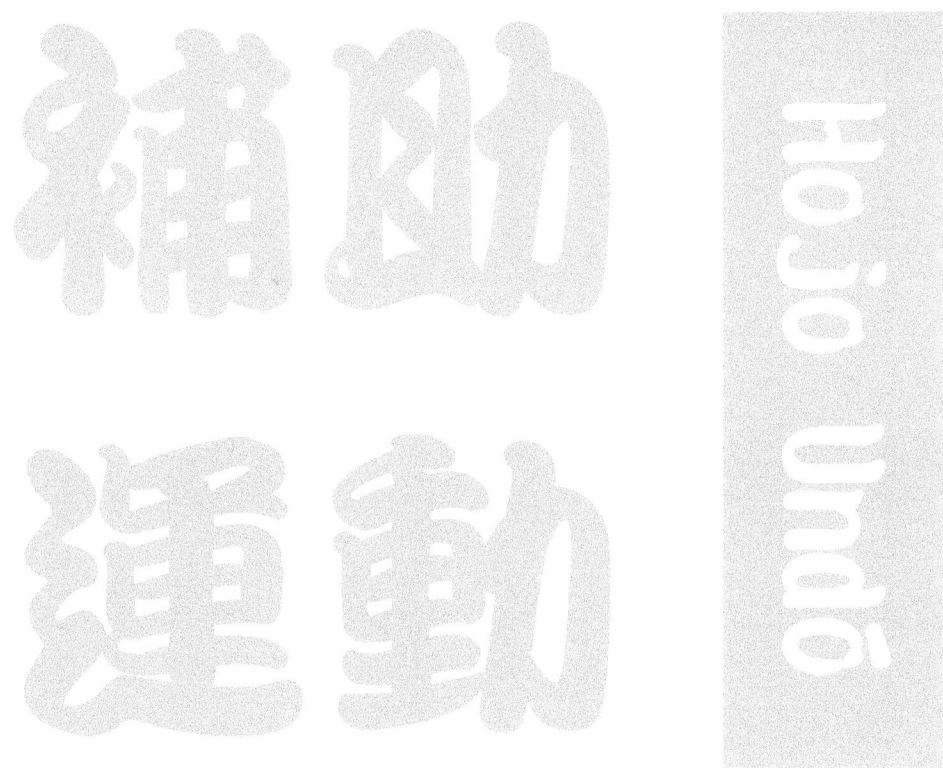

Hojo Undo (補助運動), or supplementary exercises, are essentially all the exercises that, although not part of the formal Yobi Undo, are routinely done immediately following the Yobi Undo. Unlike Yobi Undo, these exercises don't have a particular order or pattern, and the sets are usually 10 or 20 repetitions.

補助運動   Hojo Undō

Each set of squats is done in 20 repetitions, alternating sides as necessary. This results in a total of 120 squats.

Heisoku Dachi squats

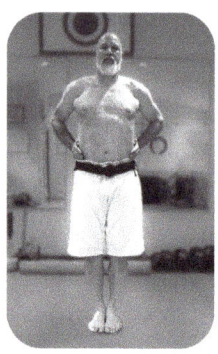 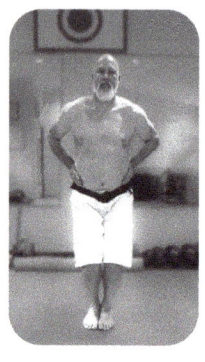 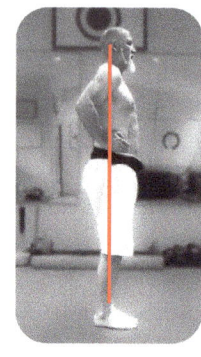 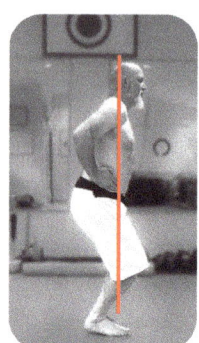

SIDEVIEW

Musubi Dachi squats

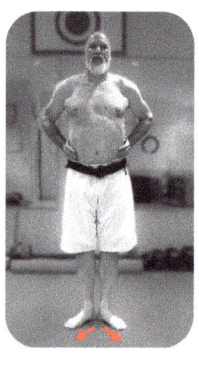 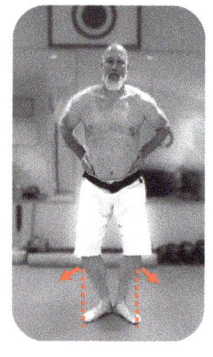 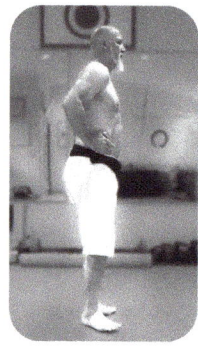 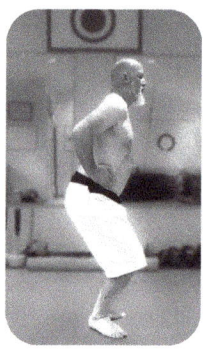

SIDEVIEW

Neko Ashi Dachi squats

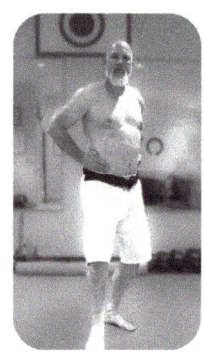 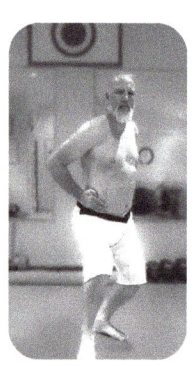 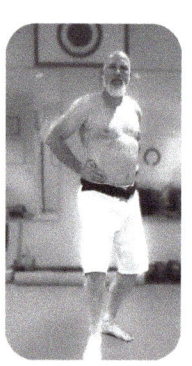 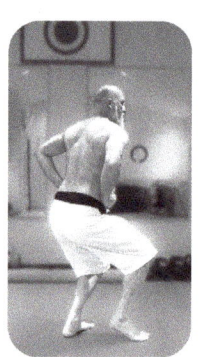

SIDEVIEW

Jigotai Dachi squats

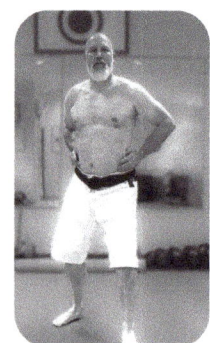 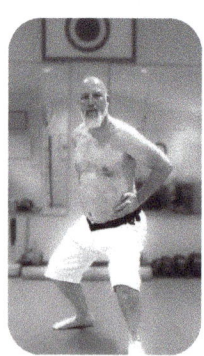 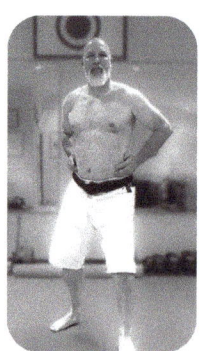 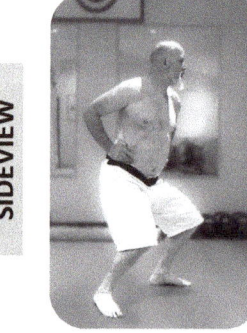

SIDEVIEW

補助運動 Hojo Undō

Squat jumps

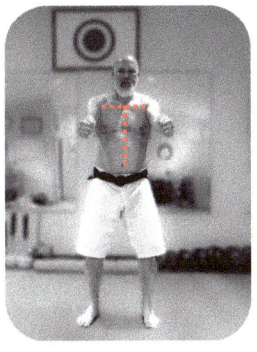 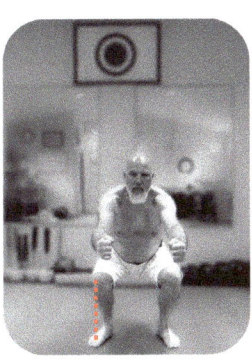 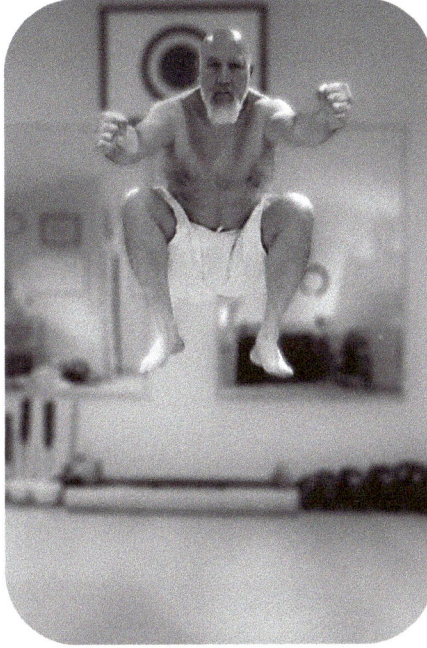 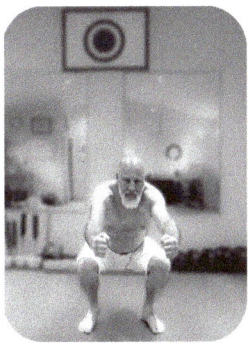

Focus on height, knees up. Push off the ground as high as you can.

Control the landing; do not stomp or make loud noise when landing.

SIDEVIEW

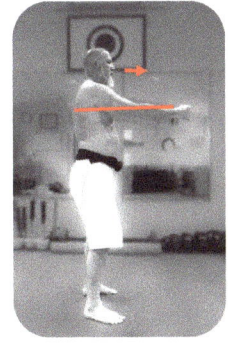 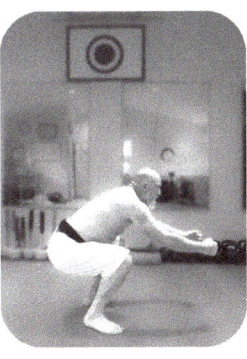 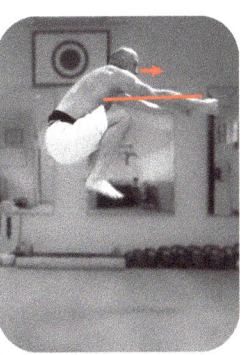 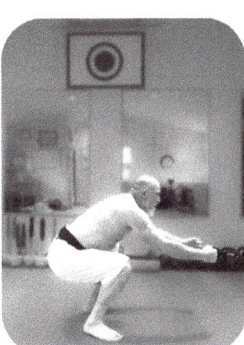

Keep your arms out in front, as level to the ground as possible, throughout the entire jump.

Hojo Undō

補助運動

Shiko Dachi dips

Start in Shiko Dachi and lower the position to the ground to begin the exercise.

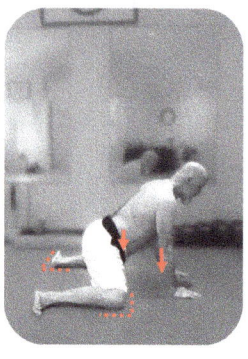 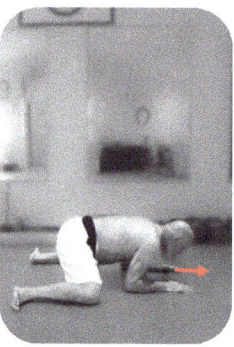 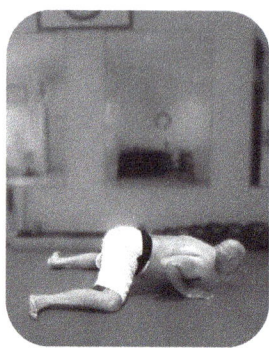 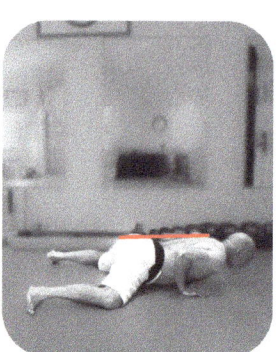

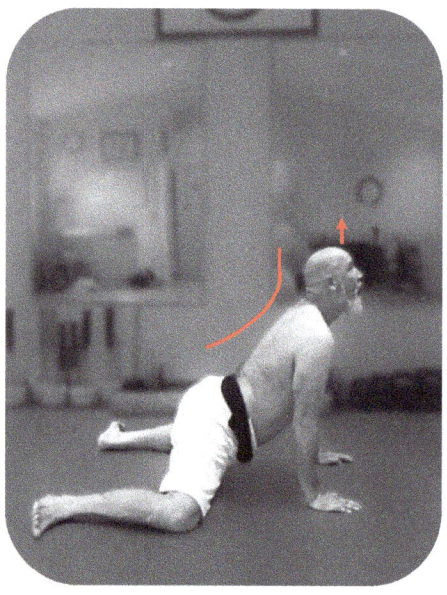 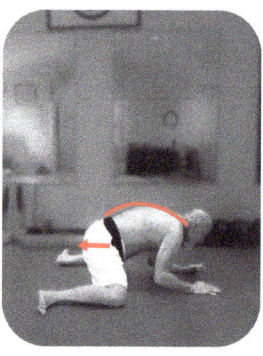 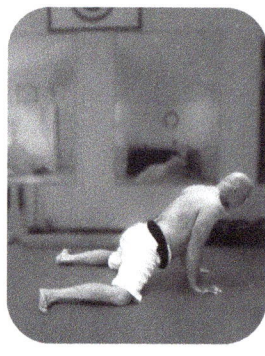 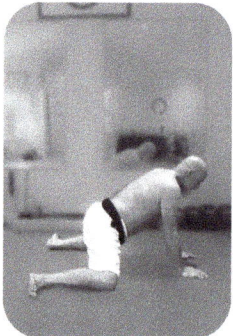

90° at the ankles, knees, hips.

Straddle dips

Essentially the same as the Shiko Dachi dips but done with legs straight and the feet as flat to the ground as possible.

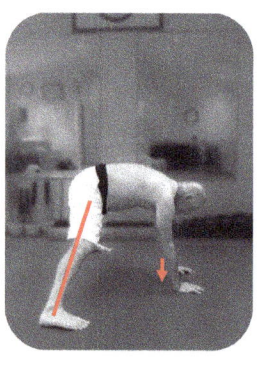 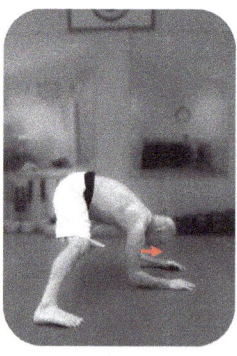 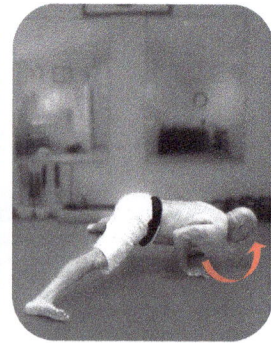 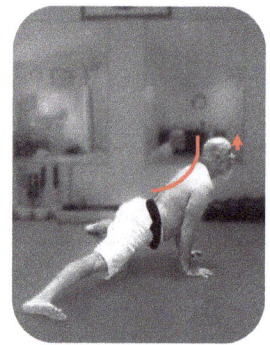 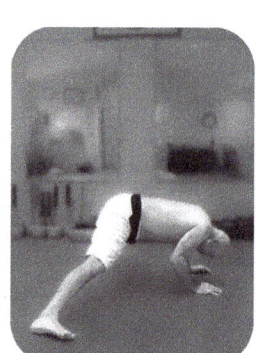

補助運動　　　　　　　　　　　　Hojo Undō

Push-up jump twists

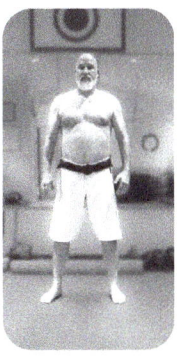 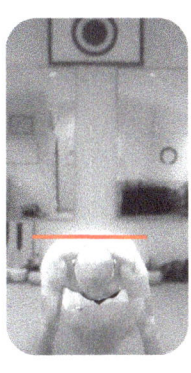 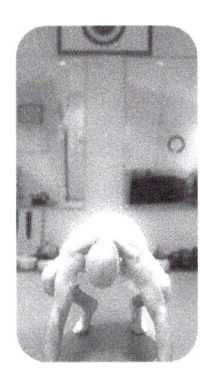 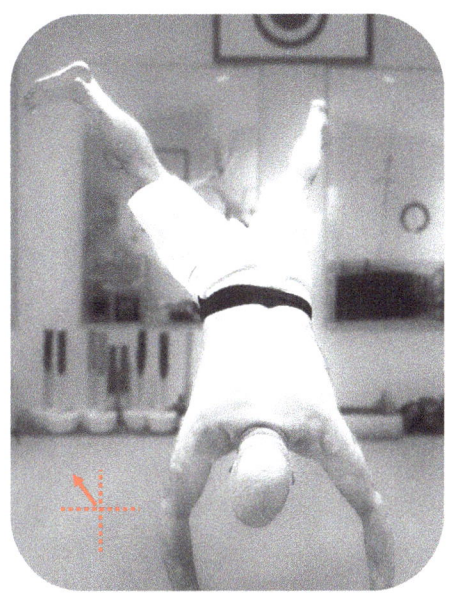

From a plank position, pull the knees to the armpits, kick both legs out as near to vertical as possible, twisting towards right, land as controlled as possible with both feet at the same time.

Raise the left leg and twist over to the ground on the right, taking most of the weight on the right arm.

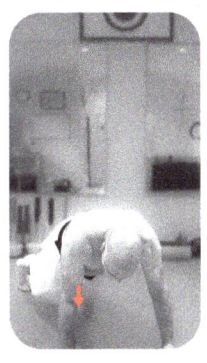 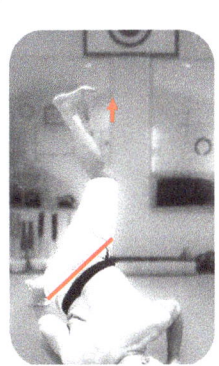 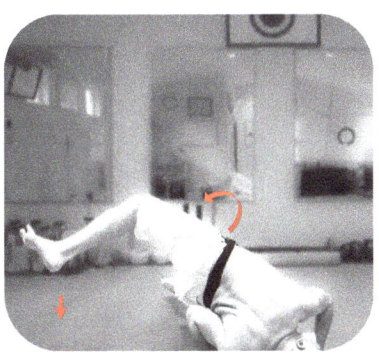 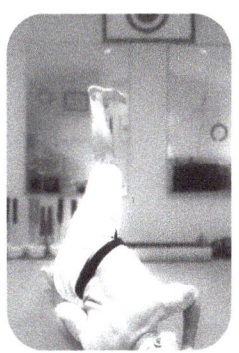

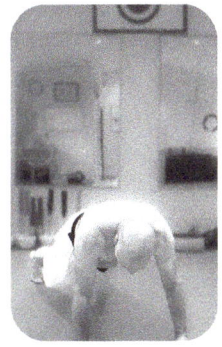 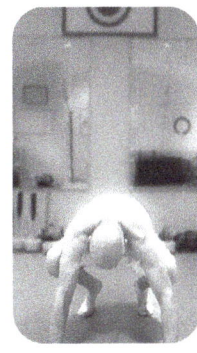 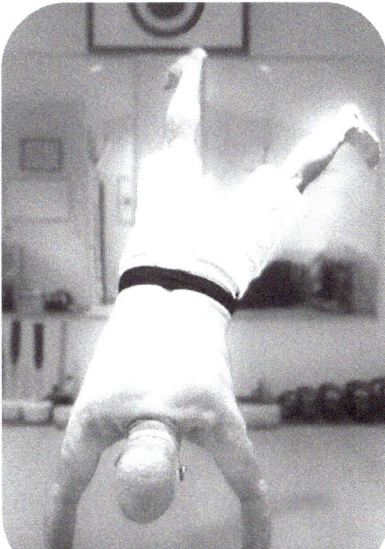

Return the left leg to the upright position, and then lower it to plank position.

In a single jump motion, pull knees up to the armpits, then repeat on the left side.

Hojo Undō

Complete the left side.

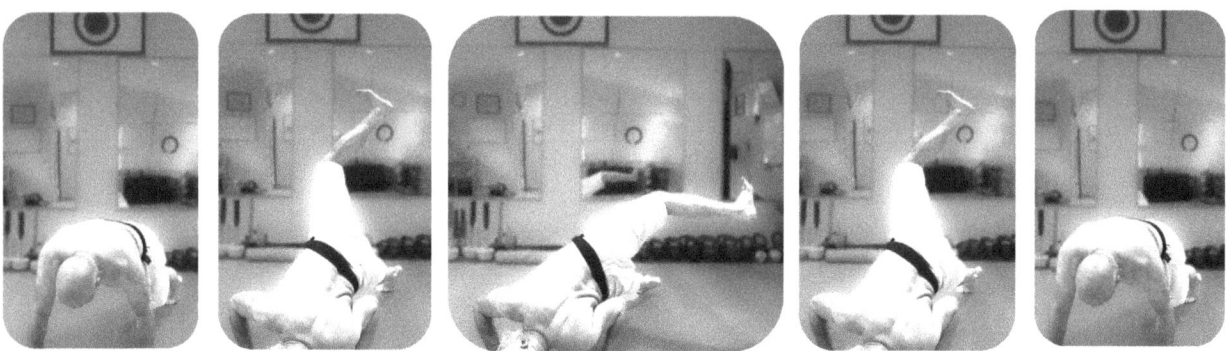

After both the right and left sides are completed, return to center and kick both legs out straight back. There is no twist on the center jump.

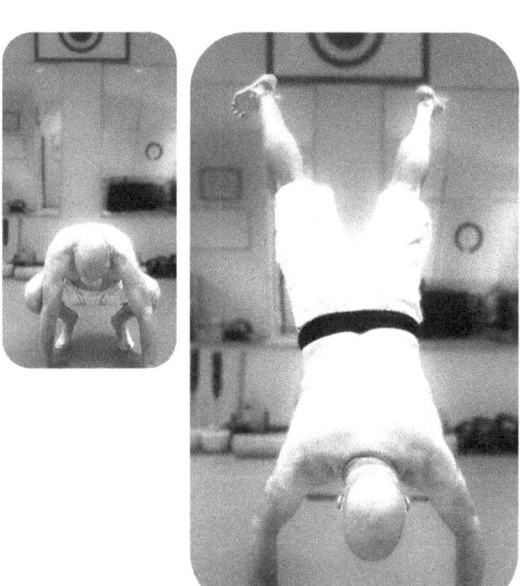

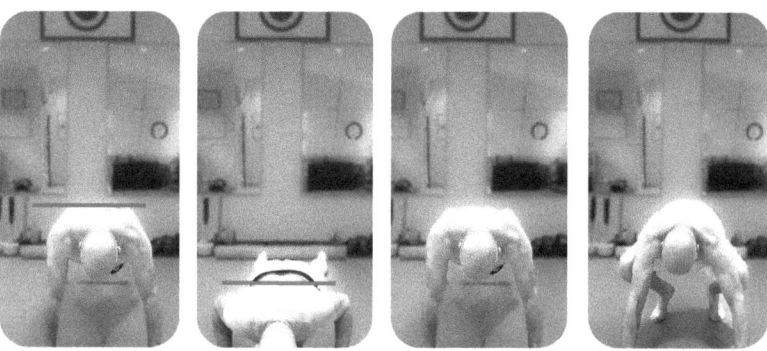

Right, left, and center make one set: the goal is 10.

補助運動　　　　　　　　　　　　　　Hojo Undō

Daruma Taiso

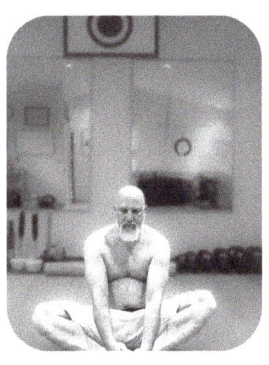 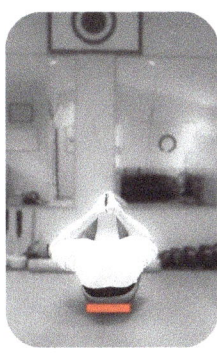 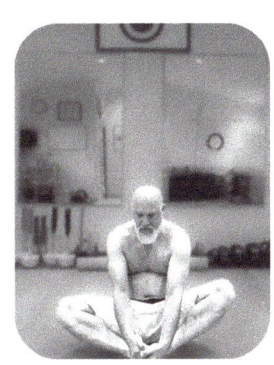

Ideally this exercise is done in lotus or half lotus position. Alternatively, squeezing the soles of the feet together will accomplish the basic point of the exercise.

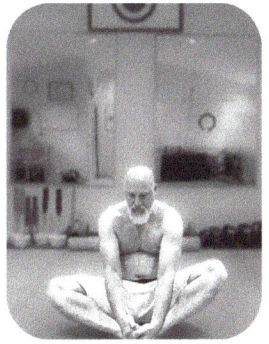 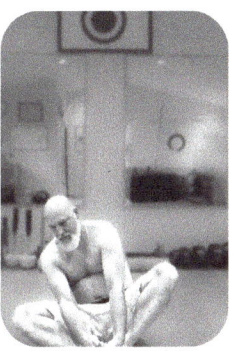 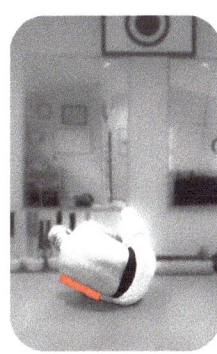 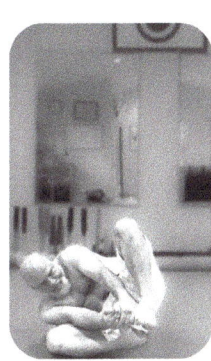 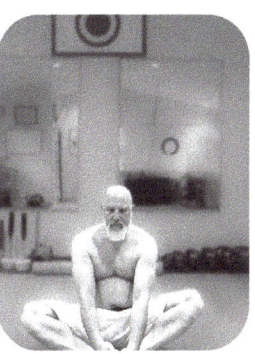

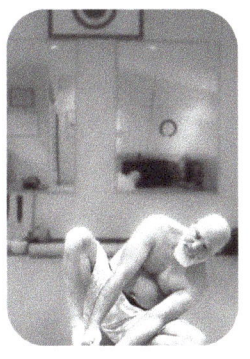 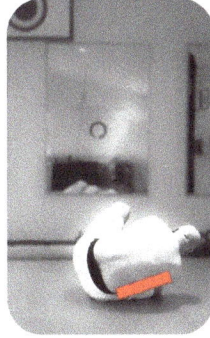 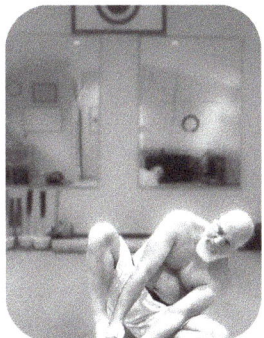 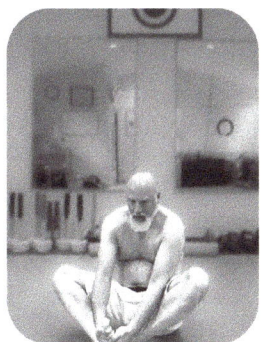

The intention is to only touch the floor with the hips, lats, and shoulders as you roll, not the flat of your back (spine). Once a full rotation is achieved, stop your momentum and change direction using only your core strength. Do not use your hands/arms to assist you. Once you return to the starting position, roll in the other direction. Usually 4 to 6 rotations per side.

補助運動 Hojo Undō

Roll back on to the shoulders, both legs go over the right, hold the position with the feet touching the ground for a few seconds, then raise the legs straight up and land in front, legs apart.

Roll overs

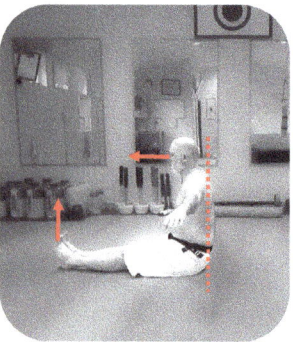 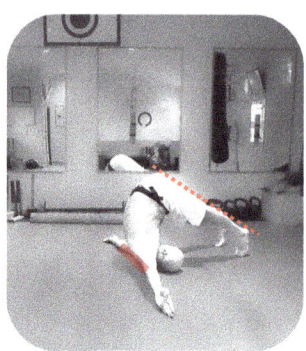 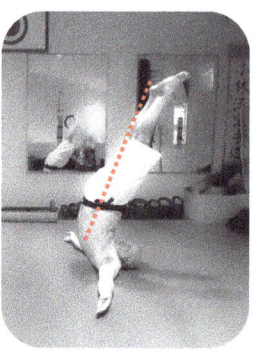

From the starting position, roll back and reach the legs to the left side, return forward, legs apart at the front.

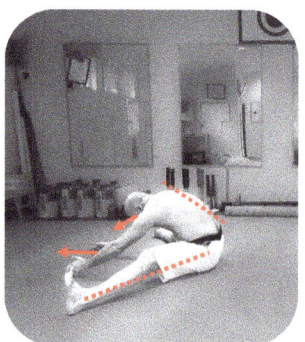 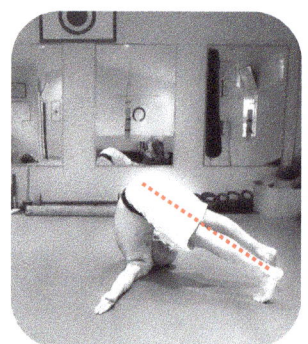 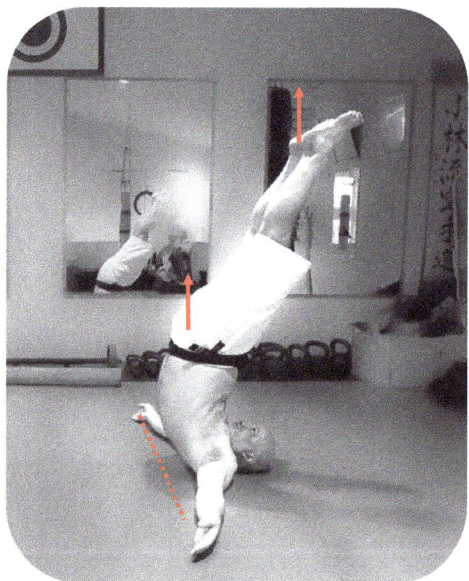

The third set, the legs go to the center and return to the front position, legs together.

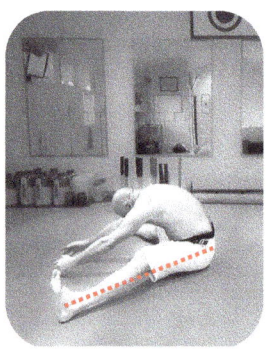 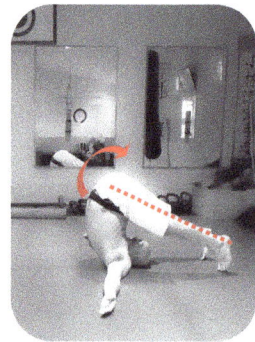 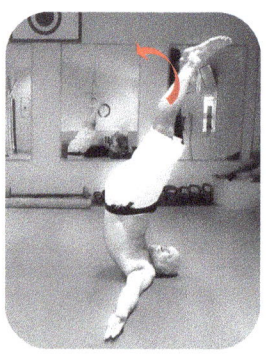 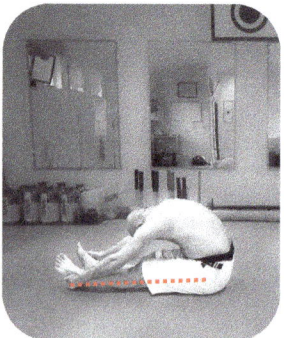

Right, left, and center complete the set; repeat 4 to 10 times.

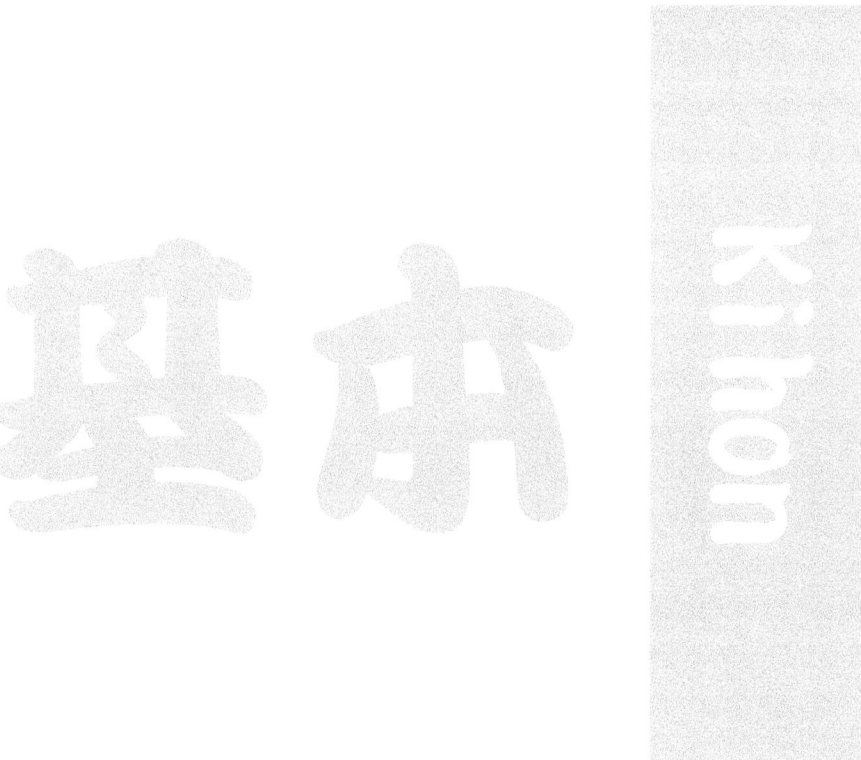

Kihon

Kihon (基本) often translated as "basics," is better thought of as "fundamentals." In other words, it is the base or foundation on which Karate is built, rather than something simple to ease beginners into training. There is nothing easy about the basics. The foundation of Karate is Tsuki (突き, striking/thrusting), Keri (蹴, kicking), Tenshin (転身, "moving") and it can, and must, continually improve. One doesn't get to be "done" with the basics.

Breathing is one of the most basic functions, but proper Kokyu (呼吸, breathing), is anything but easy and, yet, is fundamental to controlling your body-mechanics, in conjunction with Tenshin. Kokyu also plays a major role in reinforcing defensive postures, Kamae (構え).

Breathing needs to match the technique or movement. If the body is expanding or contracting, or whether the arms are moving up or out, versus in or down, or if there is a series of consecutive techniques, the breathing patterns using Don To Tai need to match.

Don (呑)- to swallow. In the context of Karate, inhale is a better way to understand it, done either through the mouth or the nose, with the tongue pressed up against the roof of the mouth pressing against the teeth.

To (吐)- to spit out. Best to think of it as to exhale, done through mouth, with the tongue pressed down at the bottom of the mouth.

Tai (待)- to wait. Usually translated as pause, the tongue pulled back, not rolled, to the back of the throat.

Kihon

Shiko Dachi Tsuki is done either stationary or shifting the stance one position to the side per strike and then to the other. When done in a group, students will form a circle and each take turns counting sets of 10 out loud, typically completing several hundred or thousand strikes. When practicing Tsuki, we seldom keep count but rather set a time goal, such as 10min, 30min etc. When doing Kukan Tsuki (air strikes/punching), maintain a tempo of 56-62 beats per minutes (Adagio in western music) and work your way from 1 strike per beat to 2,3,4 up to 5 strikes per beat while maintaining the same tempo.

Shiko Dachi Tsuki

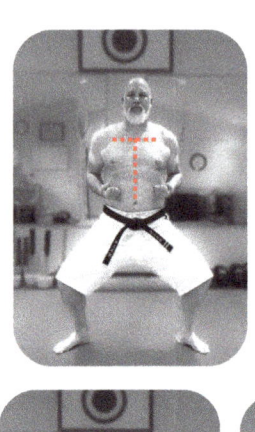 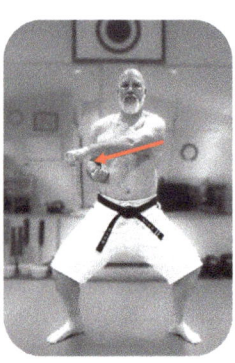 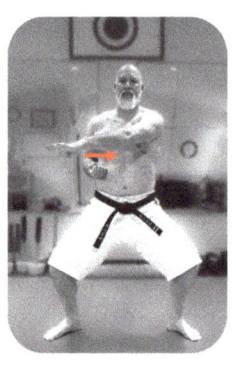 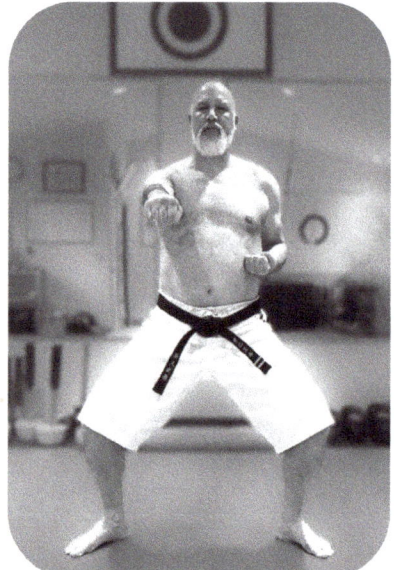

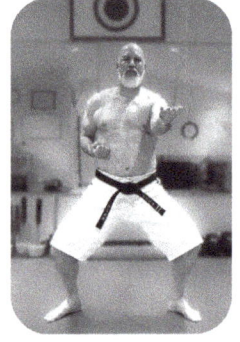 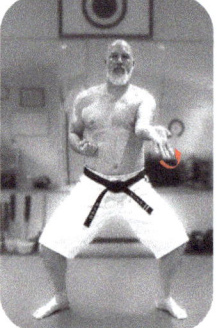 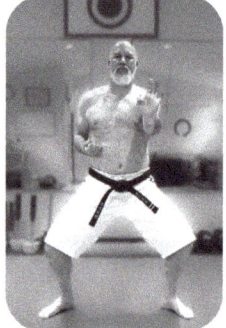 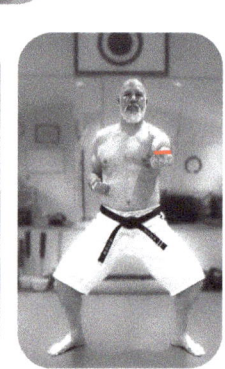

Kata Waza

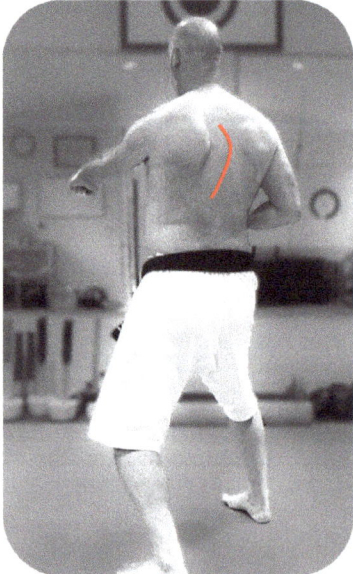

Kata Waza (肩技, shoulder technique) is key to connect the hips and legs to the fist, open hand, or elbow when striking.

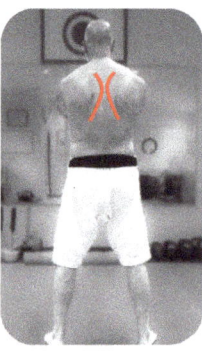 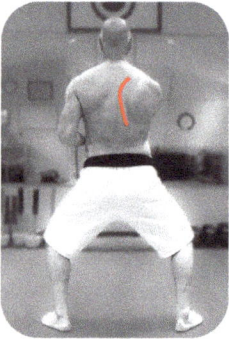 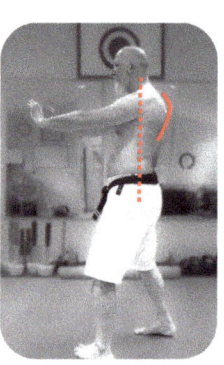

Kihon

Shiko Dachi Mae Geri is done either stationary or shifting the stance one position to the side per kick and then to the other.

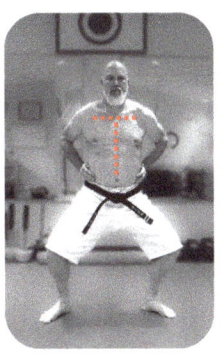 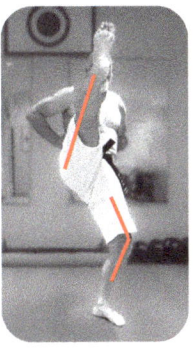 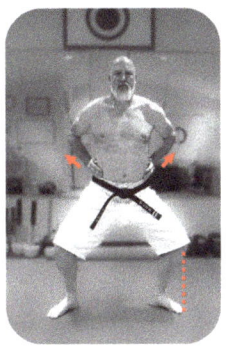

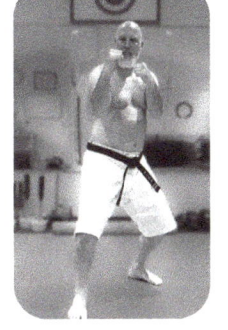

Shiko Dachi Mae Geri

Like the Tsuki practice, when doing Keri in a group, students will form a circle and each take turns counting sets of 10 out loud, typically completing several hundred kicks.

A progression from Shiko Dachi is to sit in Jigotai and kick forward, 45°, and sidewards.

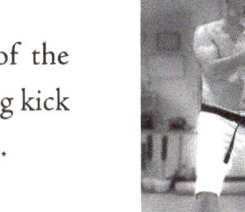

Shomen Mae Geri

Without changing the direction of the stance, the target and corresponding kick will move to each of the 3 positions.

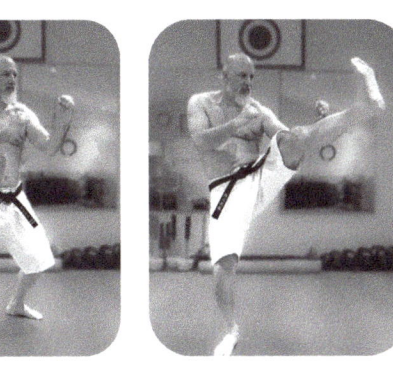

Nanamen Mae Geri

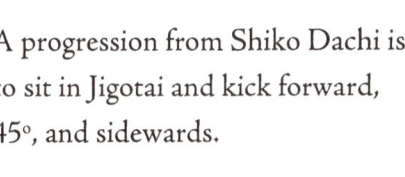

Shomen Geri
Nanamen Geri
Yokomen Geri

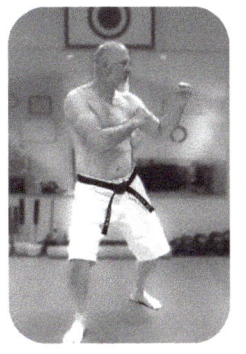 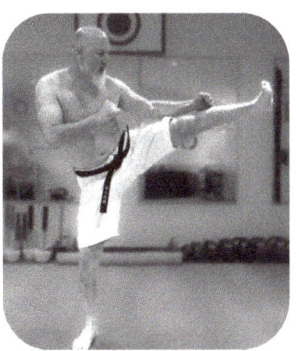

Yokomen Mae Geri

37

Kihon

Hiza Geri

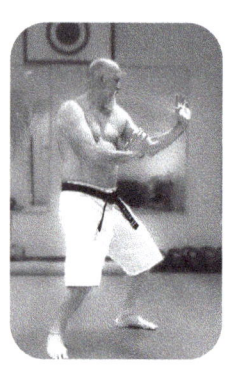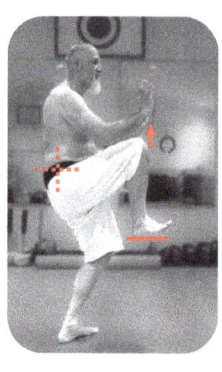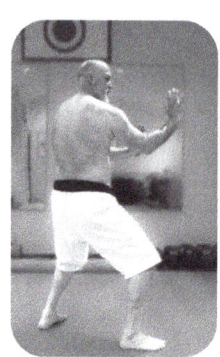

Two variations of a knee strike.

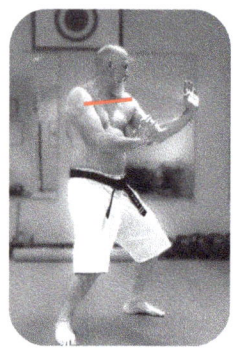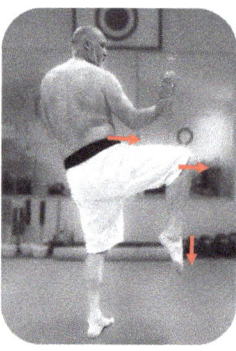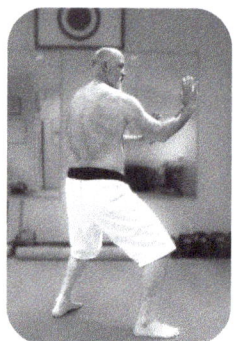

The short knee strike with the hips square, ankle at 90°, and toes up is used for close quarter combat, whereas the longer knee strike with the hips pushing the knee forward and toes pointed down is used for extending the knee kick's reach.

Kihon Dosa

Kihon Dosa (基本動作) is a generic term for all "basic patterns." We refer to the 4 sets of basic forms as "Kihon Gata," but it is not uncommon to hear them referred to as "Kihon Dosa" in some Dojo today. Other exercises that we group under the more general term of Kihon Dosa are 5 sets of Neko Ashi Tenshin and Sanchin Gata.

Note: "Sanchin Gata" should not to be confused with Sanchin done in Goju-ryu or Uechi-ryu. At the Onaga Dojo, Sanchin Gata is a training pattern that happens to be done in Sanchin Dachi and simply borrows the name of the stance to describe the pattern.

転身/寄り足   Tenshin/Yoriashi

Tenshin (転身) and Yori Ashi (寄り足) are related concepts but should not be confused. Yori (寄り) means to close a gap, to get closer, so, when combined with Ashi, or leg, one should think of getting the feet or legs closer to the opponent. In English we usually say "shuffle" to distinguish it from "stepping," in other words getting the foot that is already closest to the opponent even closer. Shuffling preserves the relative position of the feet and pulls one towards the opponent, which is different from stepping. Stepping causes the relative position of the feet to switch, resulting in the "other" foot or leg now being closer to the opponent.

Tenshin is less about the feet, but has more to do with the body. The word Tenshin literally means to "change" and is commonly used in Japanese when referring to changing an opinion, or the status of a task (for example, from started to completed). In the context of Karate, it means to change the body, either moving it from one location to another, or alternating the side that is in front, as in walking, where right and left sides alternate. Sometimes people conflate Tenshin with Taisabaki (体捌き), which would translate more closely as "body work." Tenshin is a very specific type of stepping and body displacement related to where one's opponent is; it is dependent on whether one is exposing one's body to them or not, and involves footwork that corresponds to it.

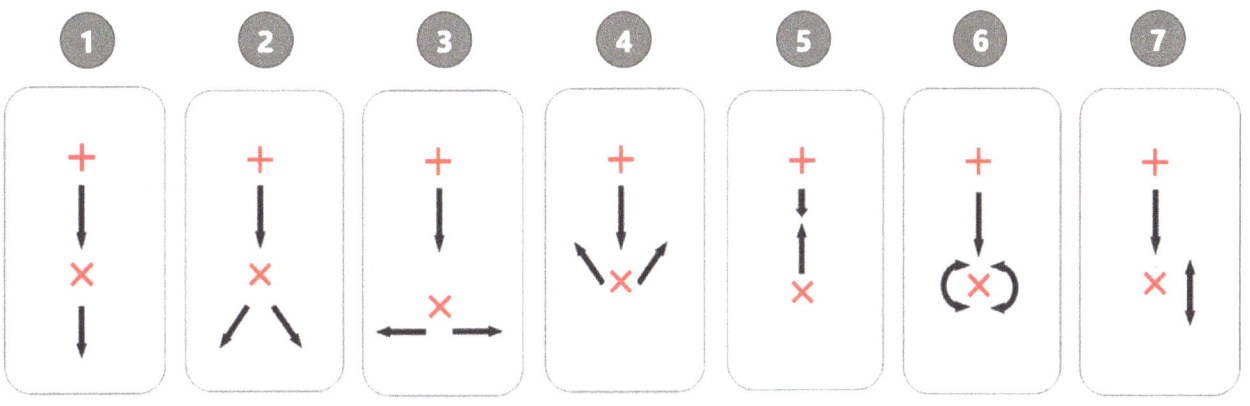

Basic Tenshin patterns can be practiced solo, with a partner, or with the Machiwara.

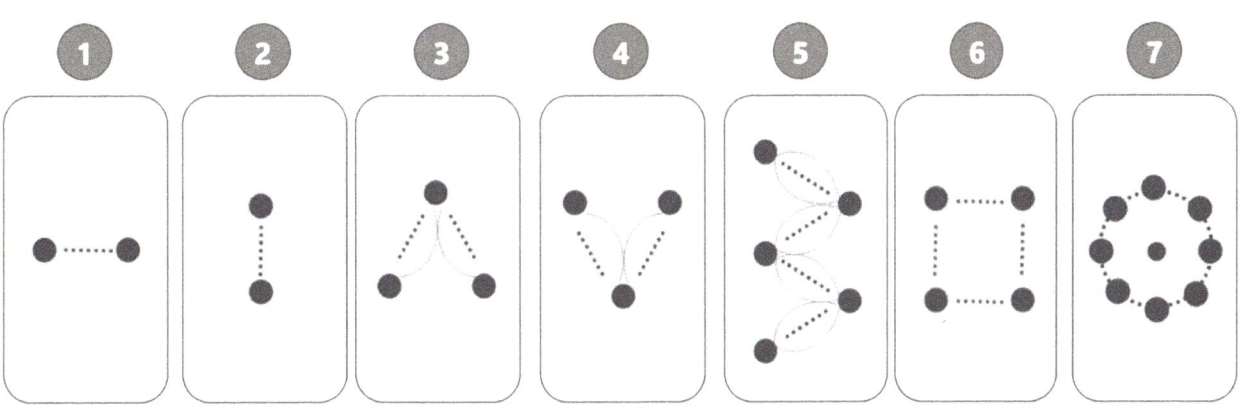

Hand contact points

手技

While there are countless methods for striking, there are a limited number of striking surfaces available.

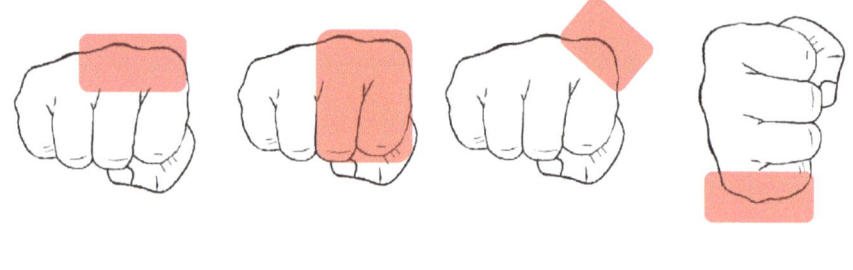

Fist contact points

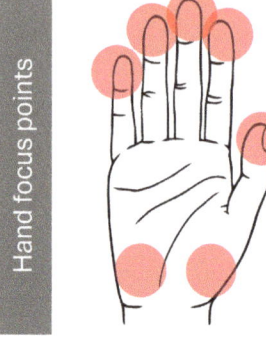

Hand focus points

The basic 7 focus points of the hand.

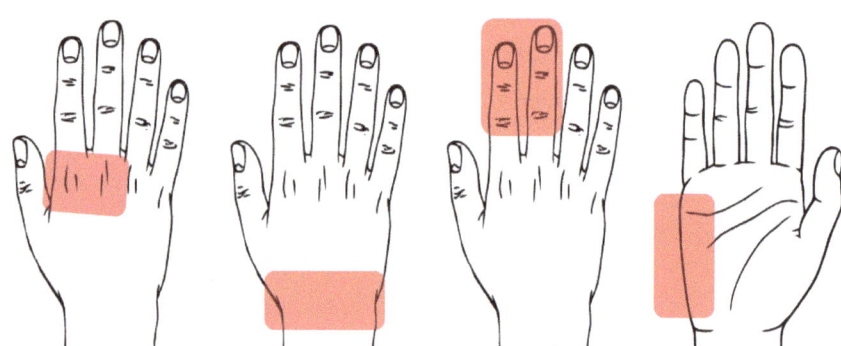

Open hand contacts

Machiwara striking areas are divided into 3: Ue (上, high), Naka (中, middle), and Shita (下, low). When doing Ue and Shita, there is the option to move them laterally. Naka is, by definition, the center point.

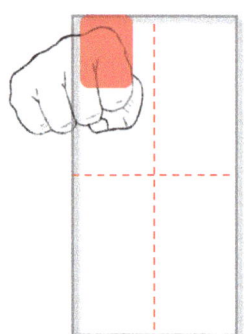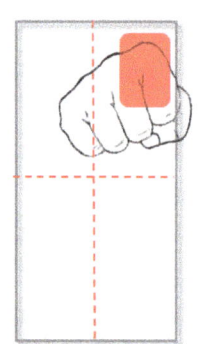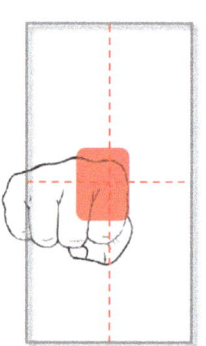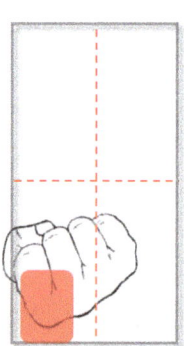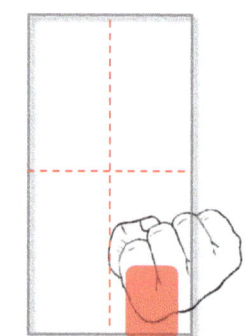

Tachi Machiwara hand positions

Most Dojo would count out Jo (上, high), Chu (中, middle), and Ge (下, low). We use the alternate reading; Ue, Naka, Shita. This is both a matter of personal style as well as a deliberate choice to not use the conventional naming that suggests a fixed position rather than a direction.

Foot contact points

足技

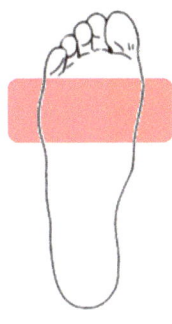

Flat of the metatarsal - used in front kick, Mae Geri.

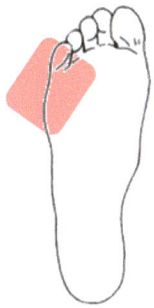

Outside edge of the metatarsal - used in angled kick, Nanamen Geri.

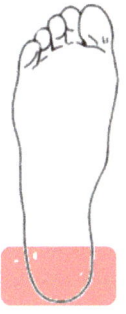

Heel - used in side-kicks, Yoko Geri, and stomps, Fumikomi Geri.

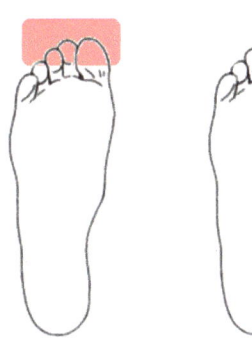

Toes - used in front-kicks, Tsumasaki Geri.

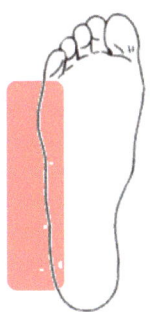

Outside edge - used in side-kicks, Yoko Geri.

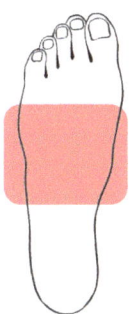

Top (dorsum) of the foot - used in rising kicks, Agi Geri.

Body Position

体位

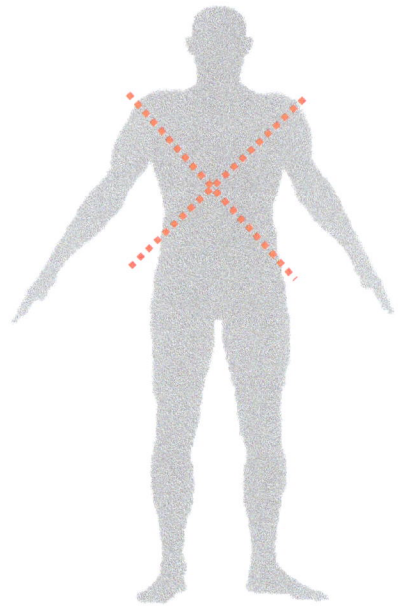

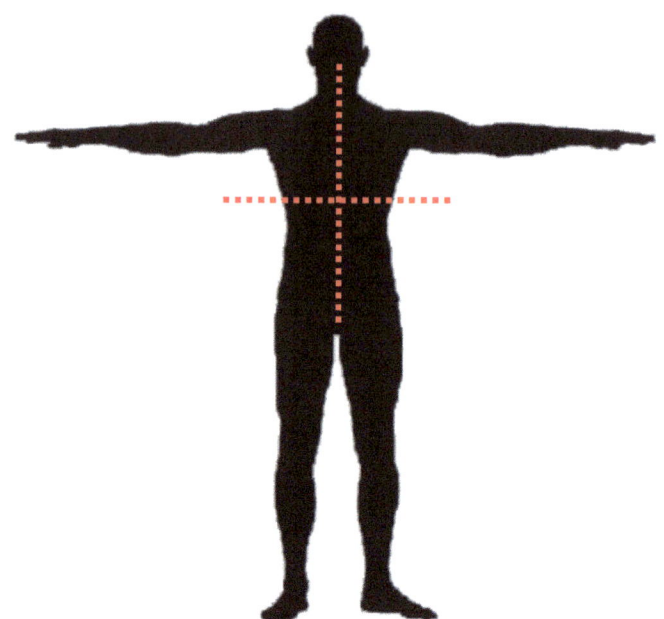

When considering one's own defensive posture we think about the angles rather than verticals.

Always consider your opponent in quadrants, with each section containing a "weapon" arm or leg.

Understanding how to think about the defensive position, as well as the likely attack, allows you to reduce the number of options to consider and eliminate the need to process large quantities of information in real time.

You should be able to choose between two options, not 4 or 6, and certainly not an unknown set of possible attacks.

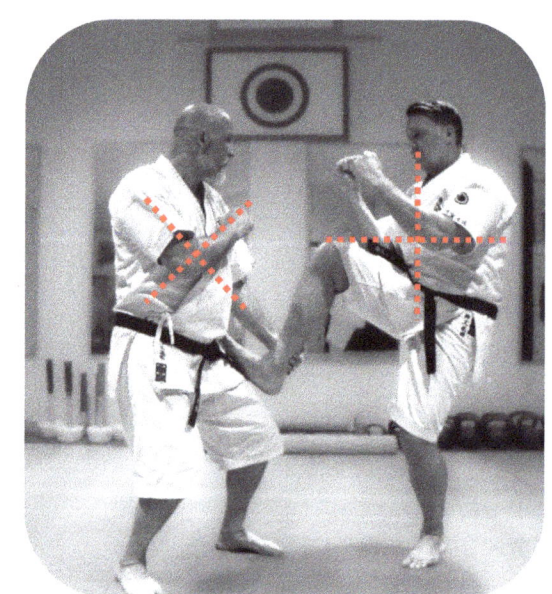

Kihon

There are no absolutes so it's important not to force things to fit "rules," but when you need a quick reference, here are a few "rules" to apply while practicing, unless expressly instructed differently with an accompanying explanation.

- If there are more than two of the same technique done consecutively in a Kata, it's important to understand what makes them different.

- The foot closest to the direction you are moving should advance first.

- Never attempt to move in more than one direction at a time.

- When moving, the most common order is Me (目, eyes), Soku (足, feet), Te (手, hands).

- Do not separate the thumbs from the hand unless actively grasping something.

- To understand your Kata, open your hands.

- Pause your breathing while striking or moving.

- Never pull a Machiwara.

- Kata needs to be correct, then fast.

- Practice for time, not repetitions.

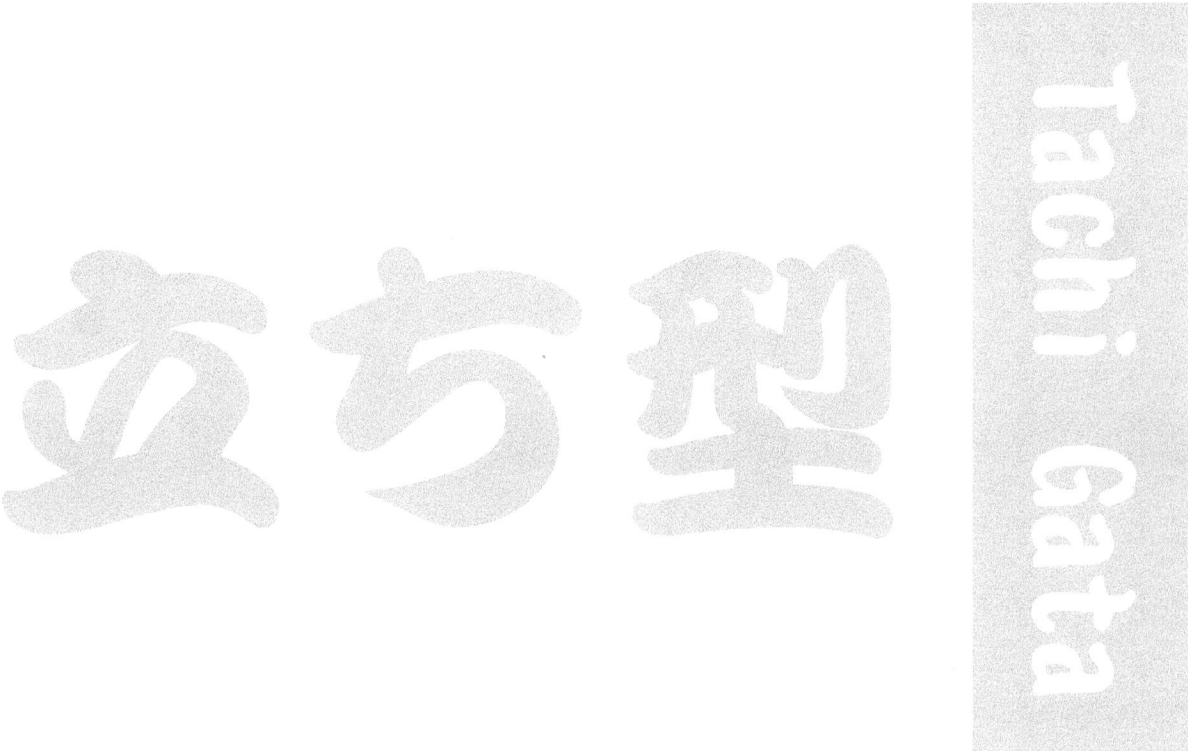

Tachi Gata

Tachi Gata (立ち型, standing positions), or stances, are the foundation upon which Karate is built. There is no way around the fact that if one is not stable when needed, or agile and mobile when it's required, that it simply doesn't matter how well one kicks or strikes.

It's important to note that although there are no right or wrong ways to name a stance, since at the end of the day, one is only describing the position, there are terms that are more commonly used than others. However, there are many ways to refer to the same position, and often context, rather than shape or size, is what makes the difference. Here are the names most commonly used in our Dojo for some of the most frequently used stances.

Tachi Gata

立ち型

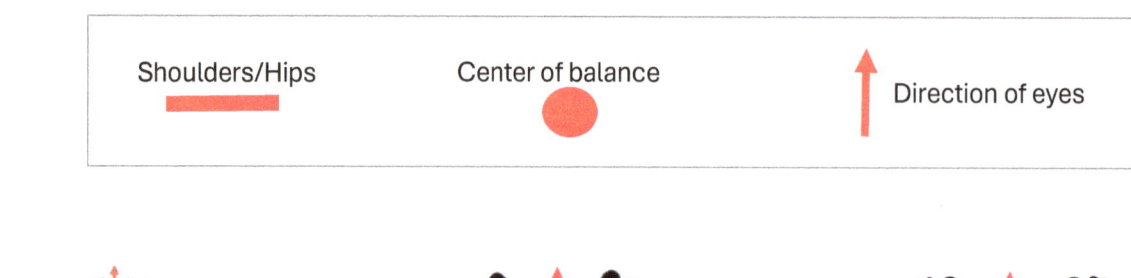

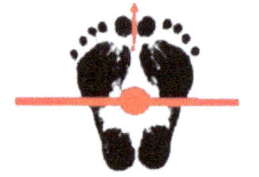

Heisoku Dachi

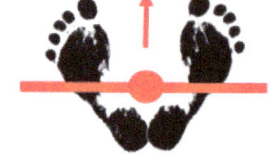

Musubi Dachi

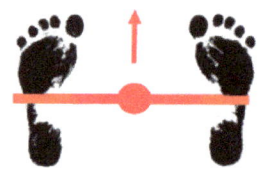

Heiko Dachi

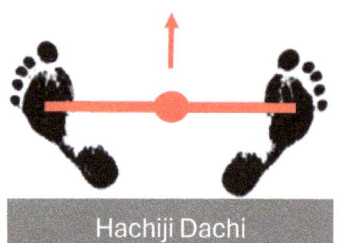

Hachiji Dachi

It is important to know how to measure and size your stance. We use the lower leg as a yard stick and typically adjust by 5-7cm. This measurement should be true for most stances where both feet are flat on the ground.

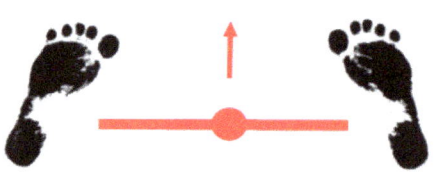

Naihanchi Dachi

When one foot is in front, the position of the rear foot relative to the direction of the stance (eyes) is generally at 45° to the eyes.

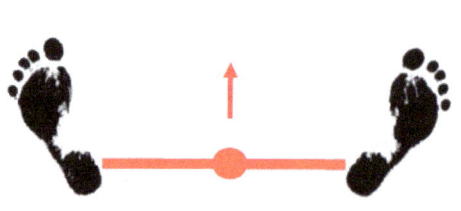

Shiko Dachi

Neko Ashi Dachi

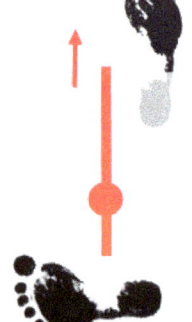

Uke Ashi Dachi

Rear foot is 90° to the eyes.

Tachi Gata

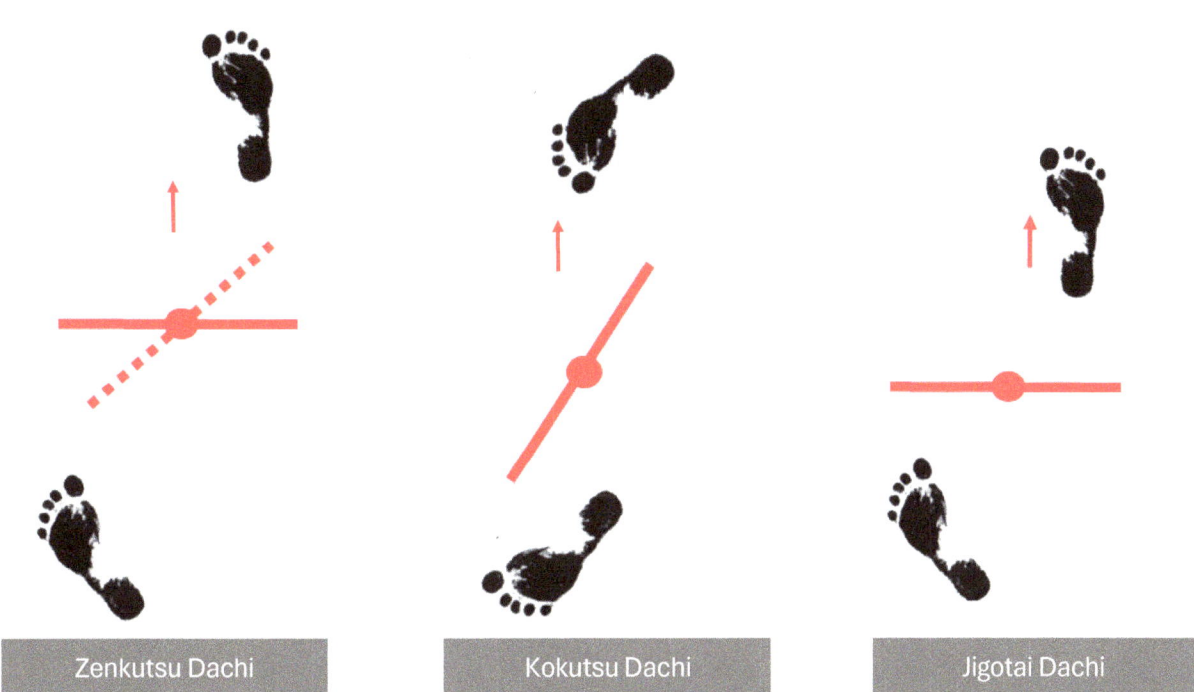

Alternatives to Kokutsu Dachi are Ukutsu Dachi and Sokutsu Dachi. This depends on the position in relation to the opponent; the stance size and shape are the same.

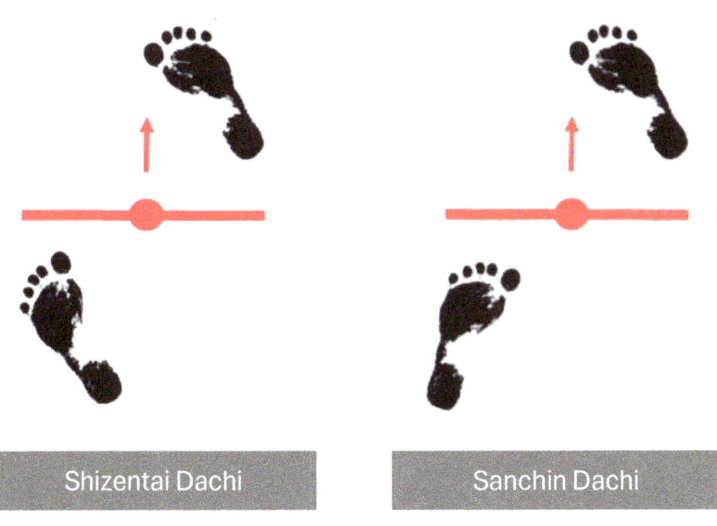

Any stance should be able to precede or follow any other stance. There should be no "dead end" stances.

Tachi Gata

Shiko Ashi Dachi.

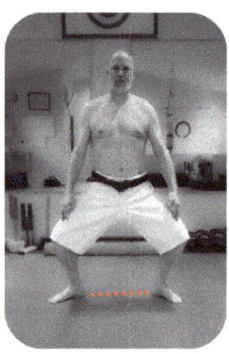 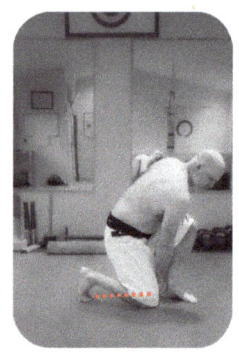

Sizing

In order to learn the proper size of most "open leg" stances, measure the distance between the heels. It should be equal to the length of the leg from below the knee, plus or minus the size of the fist.

For Shiko Ashi Dachi and Naihanchi Dachi, pivot on one foot and drop the knee to the ground.

Jigotai Dachi.

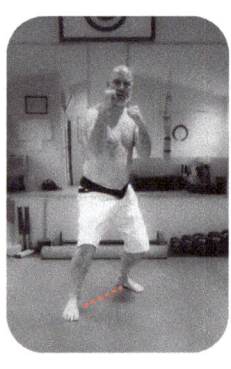 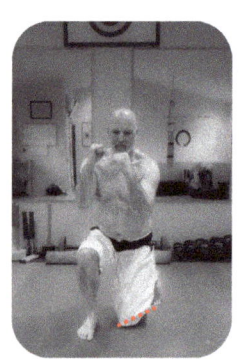

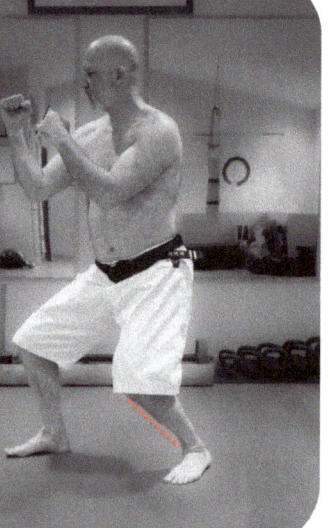 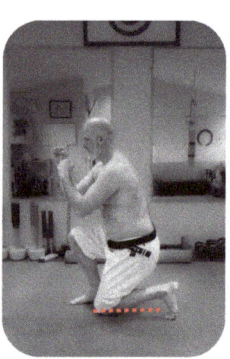

SIDEVIEW

For Zenkutsu Dachi, Kokutsu Dachi, or Jigotai Dachi, simply bend the rear knee down. It should reach the other foot, or be no further than a fist away.

Zenkutsu Dachi.

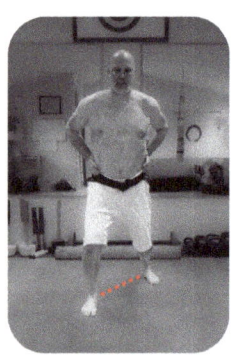 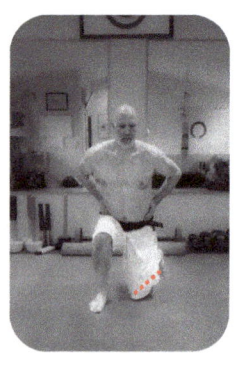

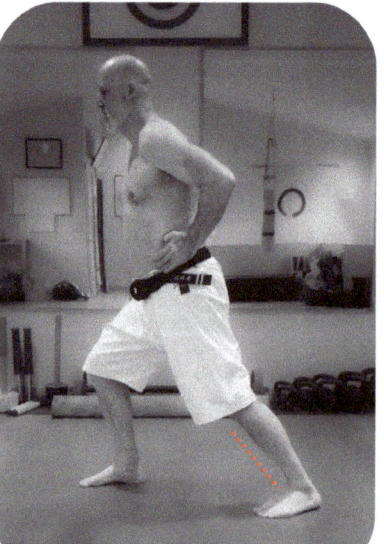 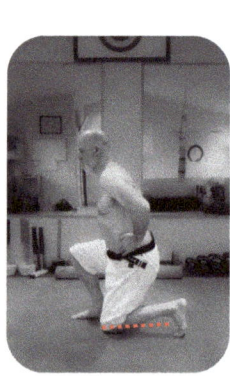

SIDEVIEW

Tachi Gata

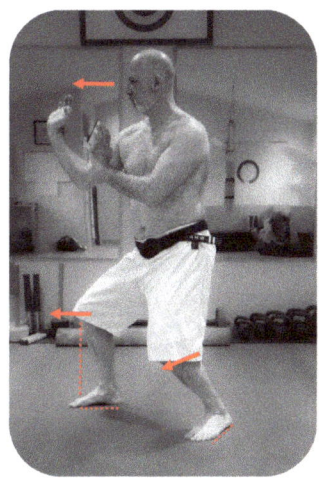

Jigotai has the forward foot flat on the ground. The front knee is bent over the toes. The rear knee and foot are at a 45° angle to where the eyes are looking.

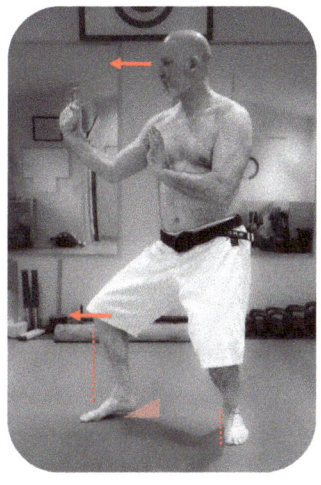

Uke Ashi Dachi has the heel of the foot in the forward position raised no more than 1cm. We usually say finger height off the ground. The front knee bent over the toes. The rear knee and foot are at a 90° angle to where the eyes are looking.

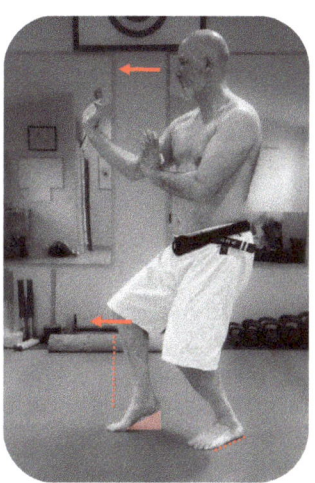

Neko Ashi Dachi has the heel of the forward foot raised approximately 7cm. Usually referred to as 1 fist height. The front knee is bent over the toes. The rear knee and foot are at 45° angle to where the eyes are looking.

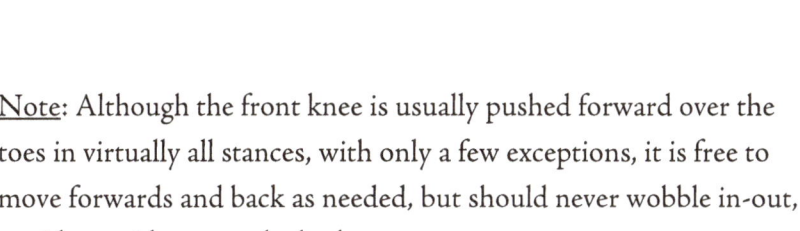

Note: Although the front knee is usually pushed forward over the toes in virtually all stances, with only a few exceptions, it is free to move forwards and back as needed, but should never wobble in-out, or side-to-side across the body.

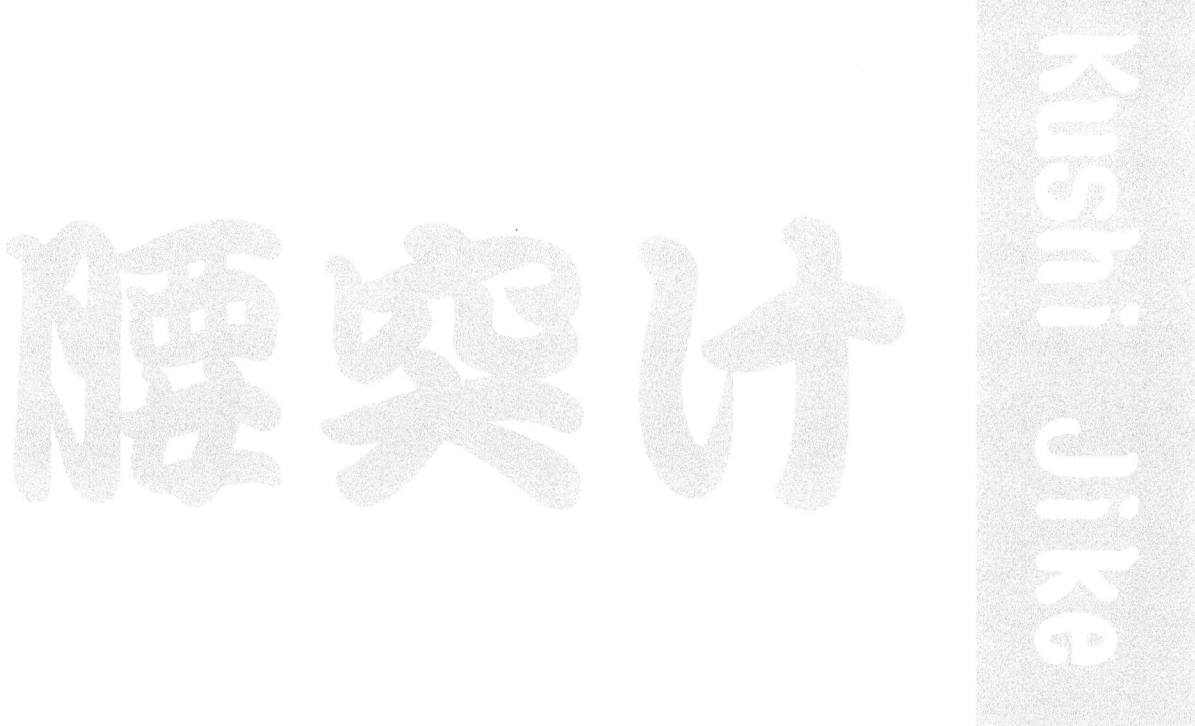

Kushi Jike

Kushi (腰), the Okinawan reading of the Japanese Koshi, is most easily understood to mean hips. The hips are part of Gammaku, the general term used in Okinawan Karate to refer to the body mechanics used for generating power using the mid-section of the body, from just below the groin, including the hips, and the abdomen, up to just below the chest.

In the Shinjinbukan, there are seven fundamental ways to use the hips. As a result, we break down the general term Gammaku into 7 Kushi Jike, or seven hip thrusts.

The Kushi Jike are applicable for both the arms and legs. This needs to be practiced both with the Machiwara, as well as when doing partner training.

Tsuke (突け) in Japanese, pronounced Jike in Okinawan, is a form of the verb Tsuku, meaning to thrust, although we usually say strike because the most common "Tsuki" is often translated as punch or strike. Tsuki (突き) or Jichi in Okinawan, is a noun "a thrust." As a result, one will hear both used, seemingly interchangeably, but the difference is likely lost in translation, because which one should be used depends on the sentence structure or concept being explained.

腰突け　　Kushi Jike

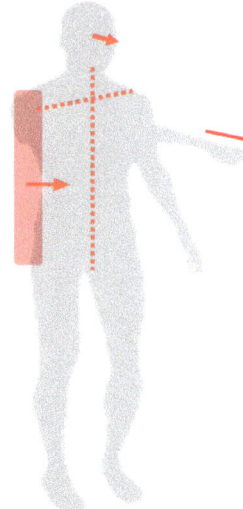

Swinging: the hips and shoulders are connected as one. When the torso swings, the forward moving side strikes. An example of this is the swinging Urate from behind the ear in Naihanchi Shodan.

Fui Jichi
swinging strike

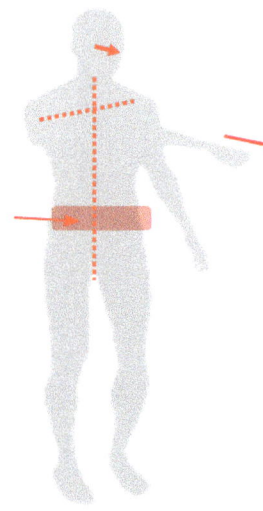

Single hip: separating the hip from the shoulders, pull one side of the hips back, striking with the opposite side. The strike ends with the hips returning to the neutral position.

Kata Goshi
single hip

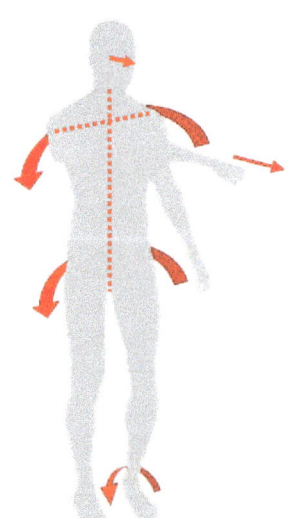

Reaching/Cranking: cranking your foot/leg (Ashi o Kuru) to generate power from your back. An example is the reaching strike in Passai no Sho.

Ufu Jichi
reaching strike

Kushi Jike

腰突け

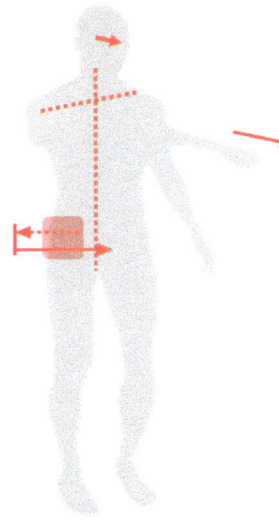

Rear contact: pulling in the striking hip to create the necessary distance to the target when the opponent is too close to get the necessary extension to complete the strike. When the hip reaches the "back wall" it bounces forward accelerating the strike.

Ushiro ni Ateru
rear contact

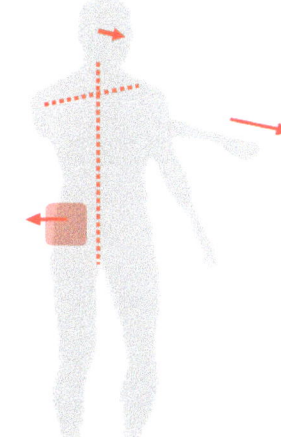

Reverse: striking against the direction of the hip movement.

Gyaku ni Hiku
reverse pull

Front contact: retracting one side of the hips when you are forced back by pressure and the distance to the target is too close. The hip will pull the strike back after impact to prevent the strike from collapsing or the body from being pushed over.

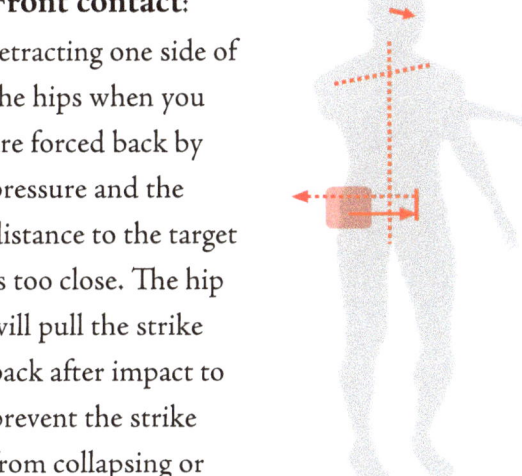

Atate Hiku
front contact

Rising: after dropping the striking side of the hips, the side that is raised will then drop to spring the striking side's arm or leg to strike at a rising angle.

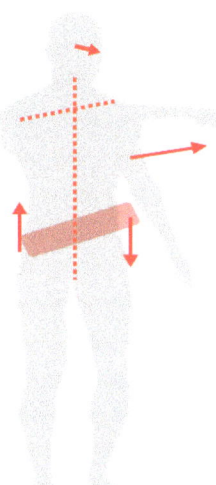

Age Jichi
rising strike

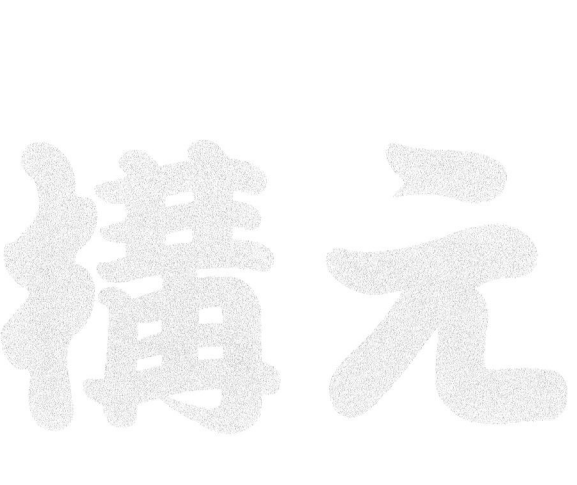
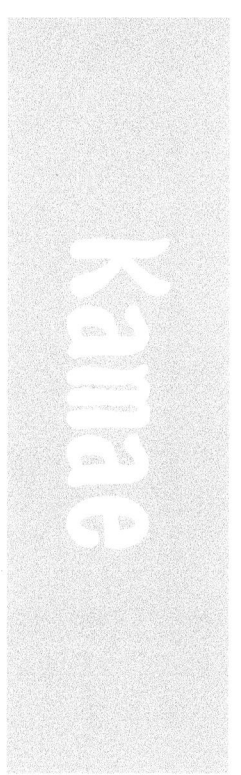

Kamae (構え), the Japanese word for posture, is probably best translated as "guard" or "ready position," or what European sword arts would call "en garde." However, unlike competitive fencing or sports Karate, we have many different Kamae. Circumstances and one's intentions and preference will all affect what risks we are willing to take to achieve our goals. There is no perfect defense and so trade-offs need to be made. It is important to make deliberate choices and understand the advantages and disadvantages, rather than being surprised by the opponent's reactions.

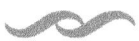

Kamae

Although there are many different Kamae, these are the most common.

Mawashi Gamae

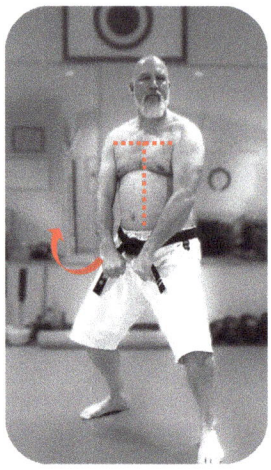
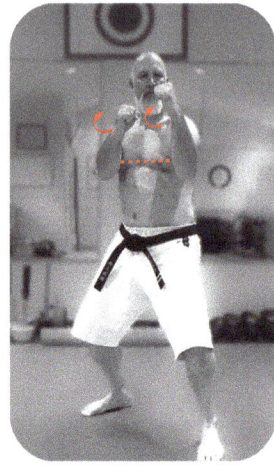
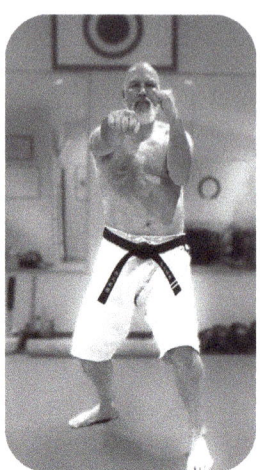

Yama Gamae

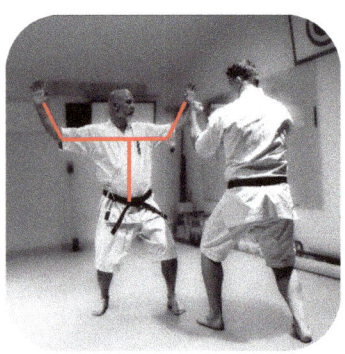
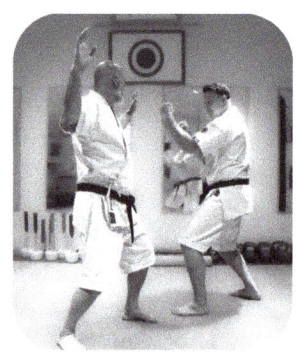
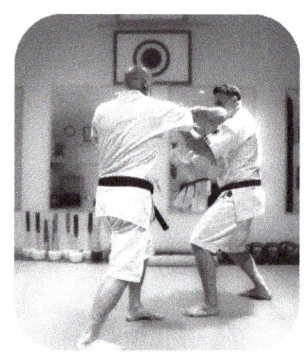

Jodan Gamae

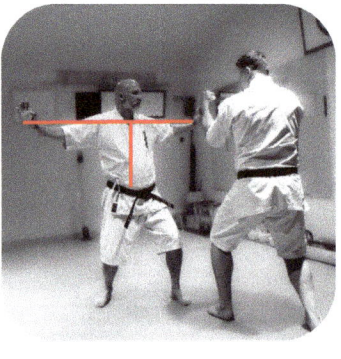
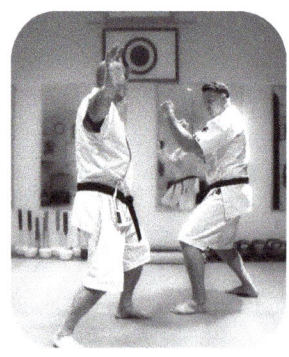
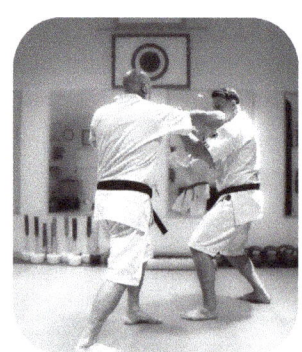

Kamae

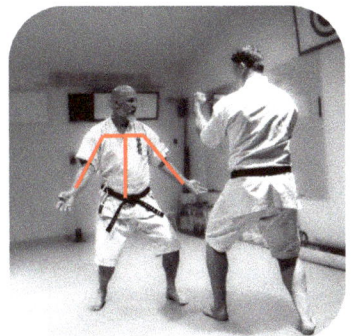 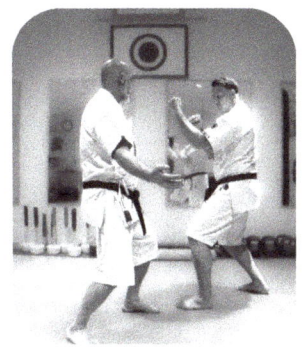 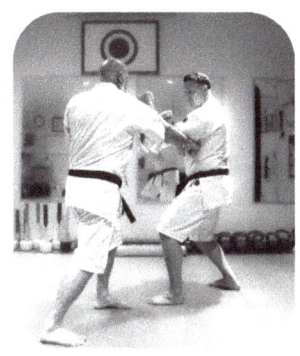

Gedan Soto Gamae

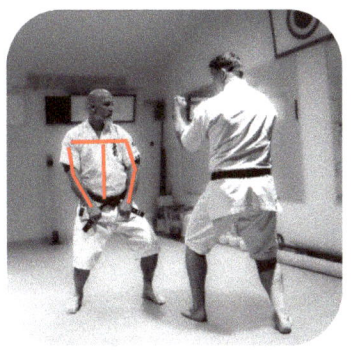 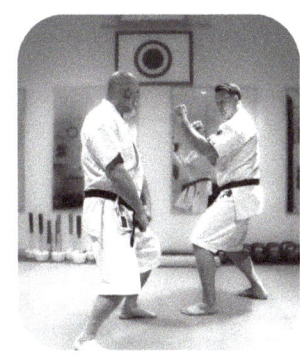 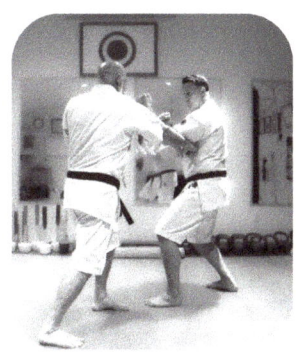

Gedan Uchi Gamae

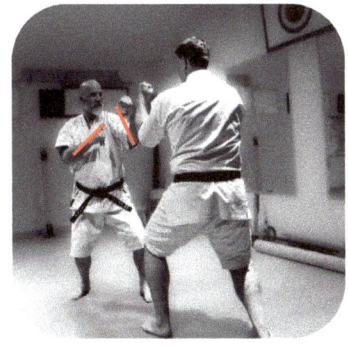 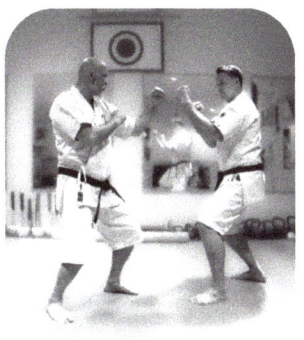 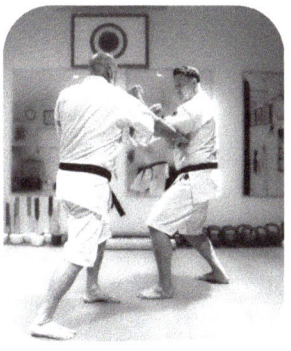

Chudan Gamae

Each Kamae is deliberately protecting and/or exposing certain target areas in order to control the options available to the opponent.

Kigu Undō

Kigu Undo (器具運動), apparatus or equipment exercises, are essentially any training in the Dojo which uses something to provide resistance, to develop strength and agility, or that corrects the technique by forcing a particular movement to follow a certain path or by adding some level of risk that encourages the student to focus on proper technique. Each tool and corresponding exercise should map directly to Karate and should not be seen as a form of weightlifting or cardio exercise. There are certainly strength and cardio benefits, but if that is the student's primary goal, there are likely better ways that can be accomplished. These exercises are specifically intended to map to movements done in Karate.

器具運動　　　　　　　　　　　　　　　　　Kigu Undō

These are traditional training tools. Other more modern equipment is also sometimes used in the Dojo but are not considered part of the curriculum.

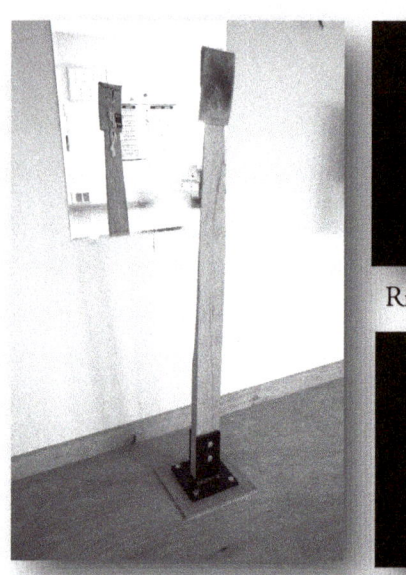

Tachi Machiwara

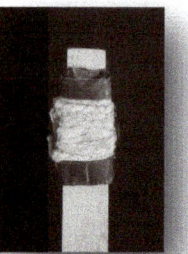

Rice straw wrap

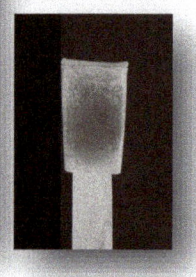

Leather cover

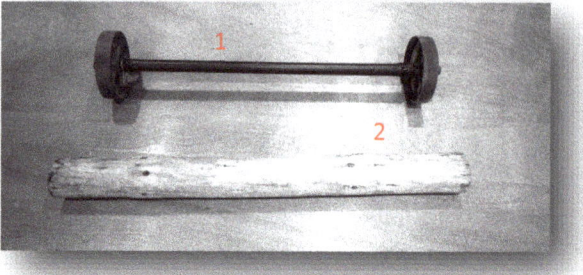

1) Tan, 13.5kg iron bar and wheels
2) Maruta or "rogu" —log

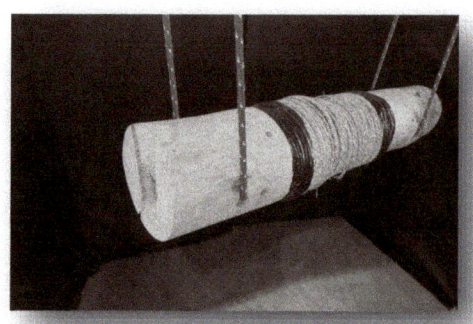

Sagi Machiwara

1— Nigiri Dama
2— Ti Machiwara
3— Hammers
4— Kicking block
5— Foot roller
6— Nunchaku
7— Taketaba

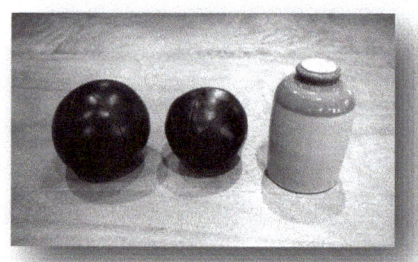

10kg Medicine balls & Kame

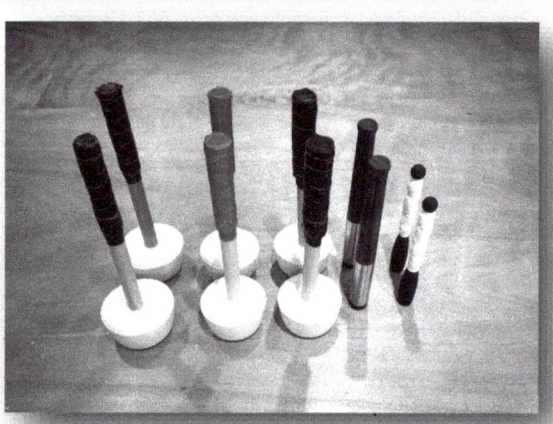

Chiishi— "power stone" traditional free weights 2.5kg and up

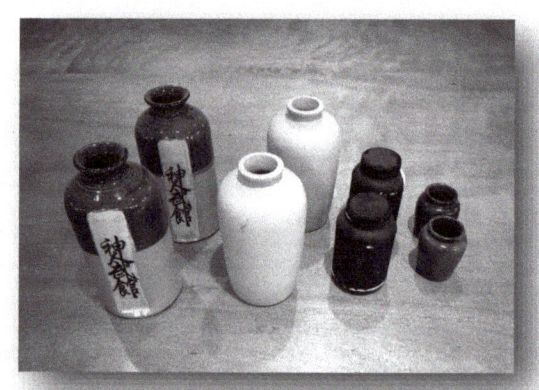

Kame (Kami) - jars of varied sizes and weights

60

器具運動 Kigu Undō

Chiishi

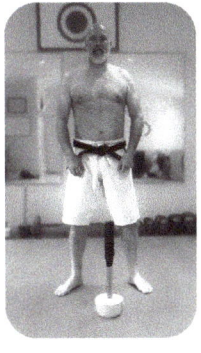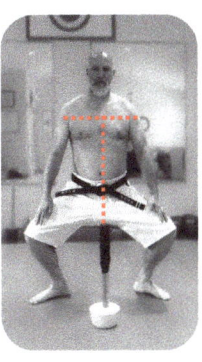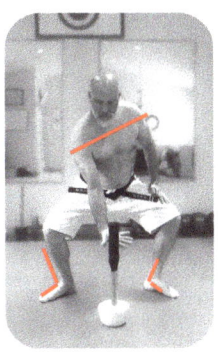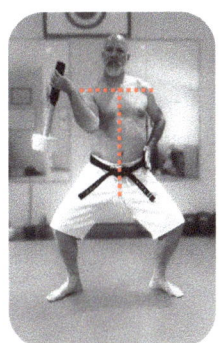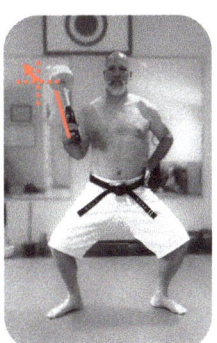

Preparation

The correct weight is one which allows you to complete repetitions without losing form.

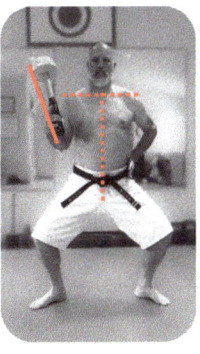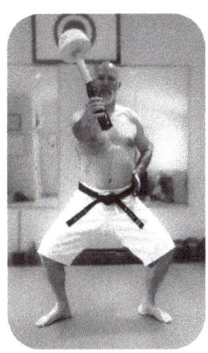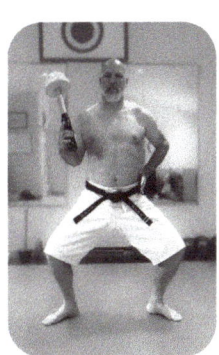

Hikite

One should select a weight with which they can complete 10 repetitions of an exercise with moderate effort.

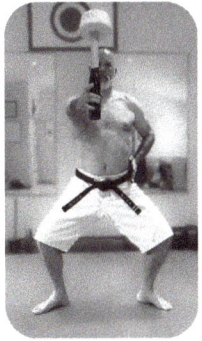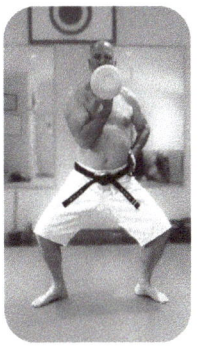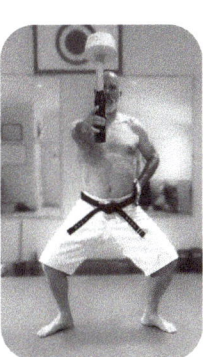

Center

The size of the grip should be large enough to prevent the thumb and the index finger from touching when holding the Chiishi.

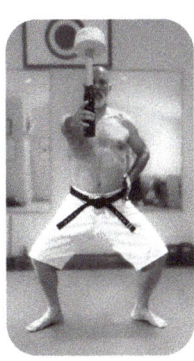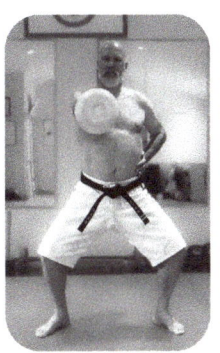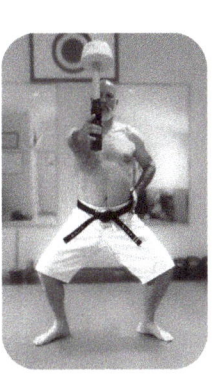

Forward dip

器具運動　　　　　　　　　　　　　　　　　　　Kigu Undō

Over shoulder

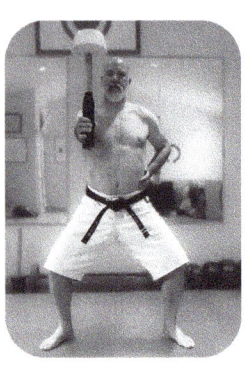 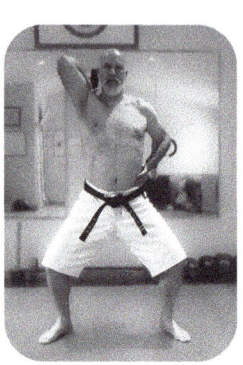 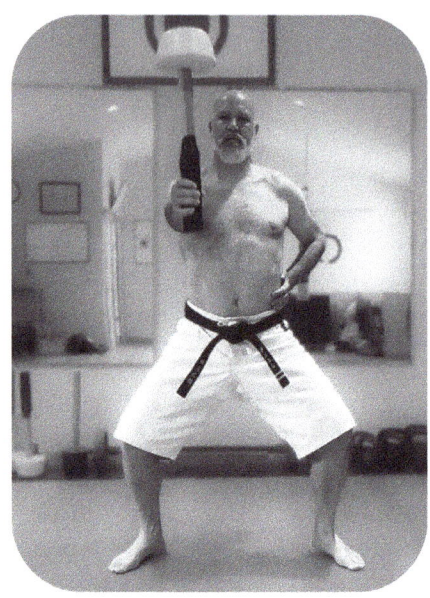

Reset

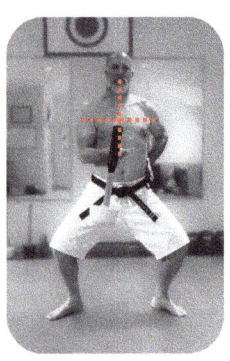 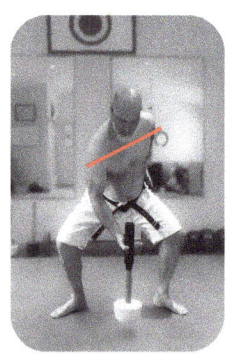 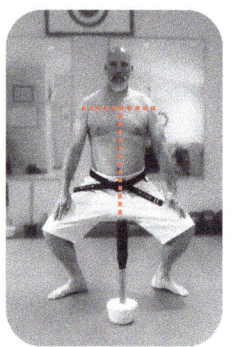

Two hands over

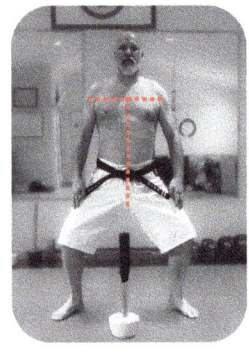 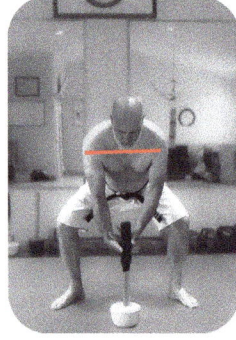 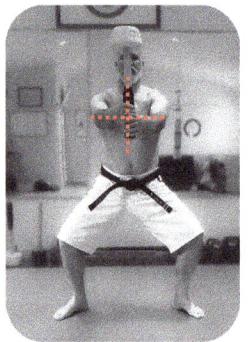

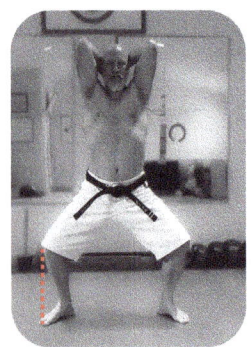 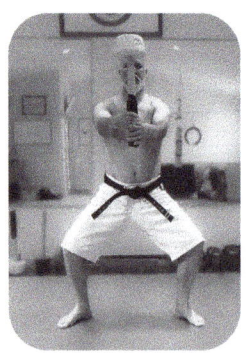 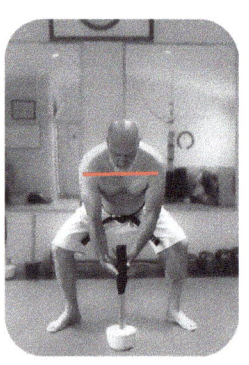

Always bend at the knees when lifting the Chiishi off the ground. If needed, tilt at the hips. <u>Do not</u> hunch over to collect the Chiishi.

器具運動　　　　　　　　　　　　　　　Kigu Undō

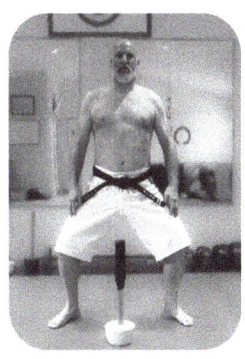 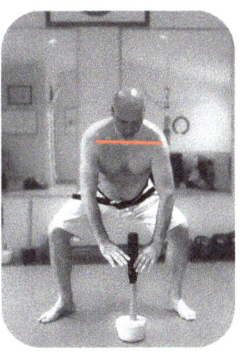 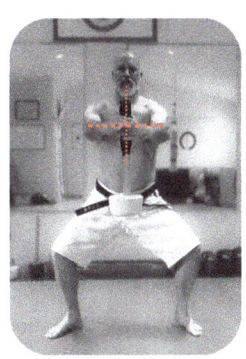 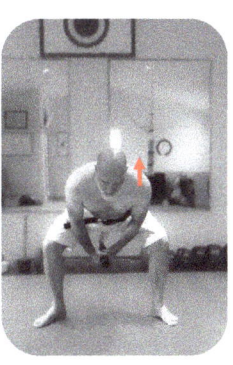

Two hands under

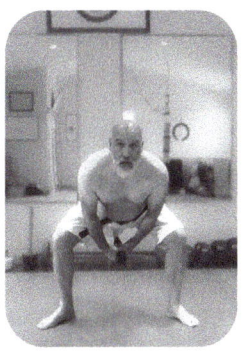 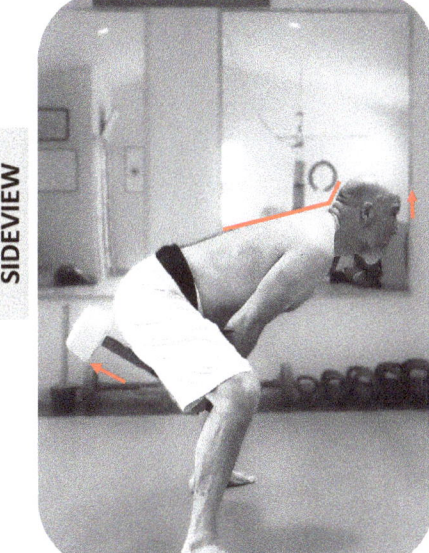 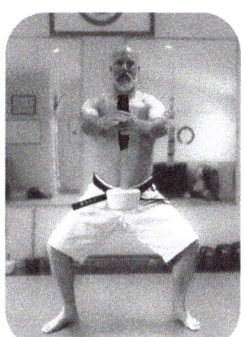

SIDEVIEW

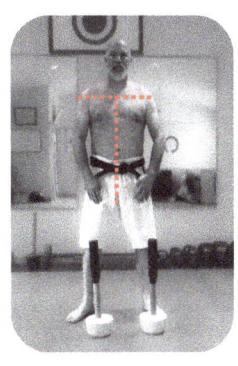 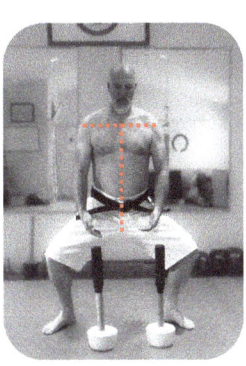 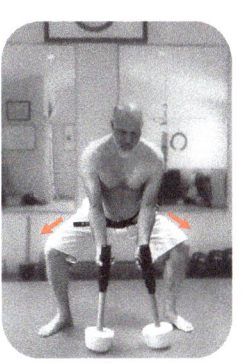 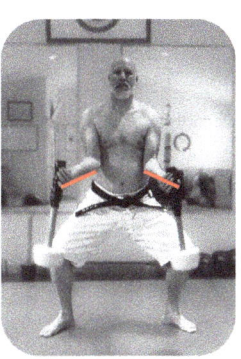

Preparation

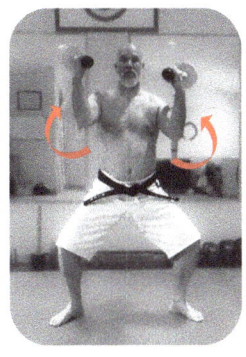 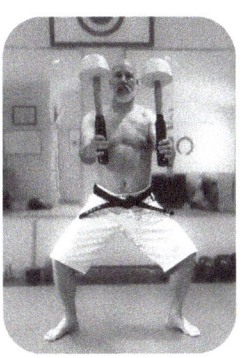

This is a common pattern for starting two-handed Chiishi exercises.

63

器具運動   Kigu Undō

Preparation

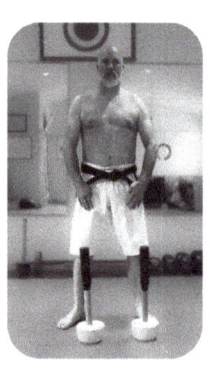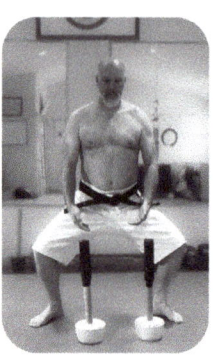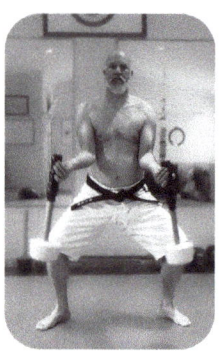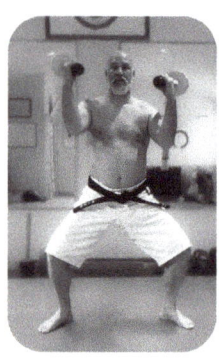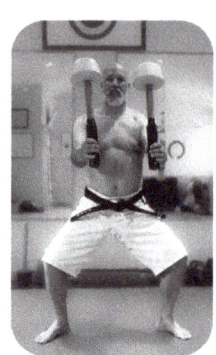

Hikite

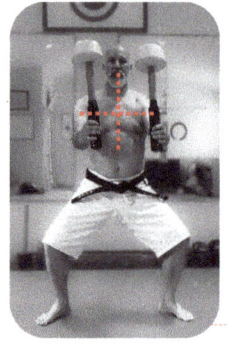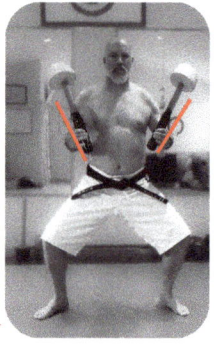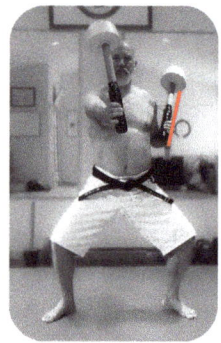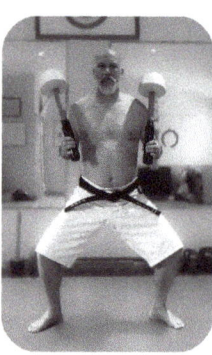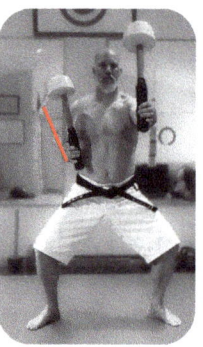

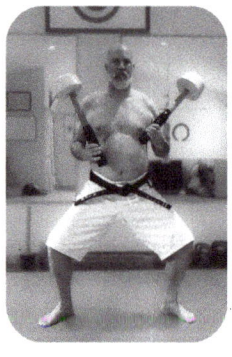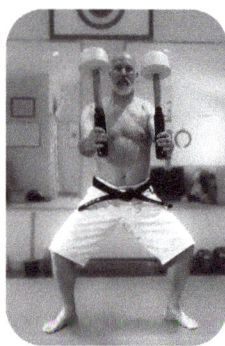

When doing two-handed exercises, the stationary arm is as important as the moving arm and the stance.

Focus on proper stances, breathing, and Chinkuchi.

Over shoulder

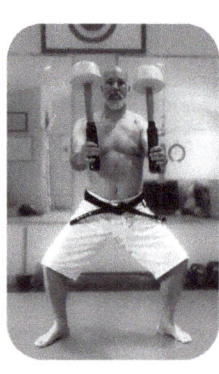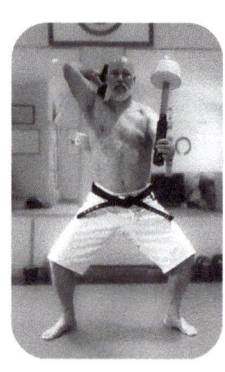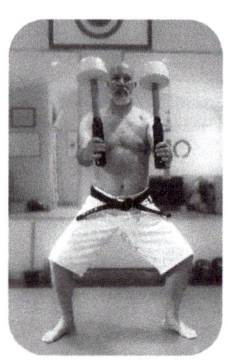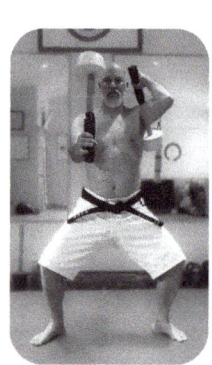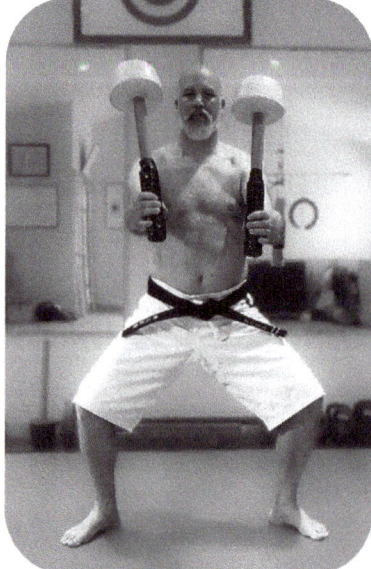

器具運動　　　　　　　　　　　　　　　　　　Kigu Undō

The moving arm is the same as single-handed Chiishi, but there is also focus on the retractor in the two-handed version.

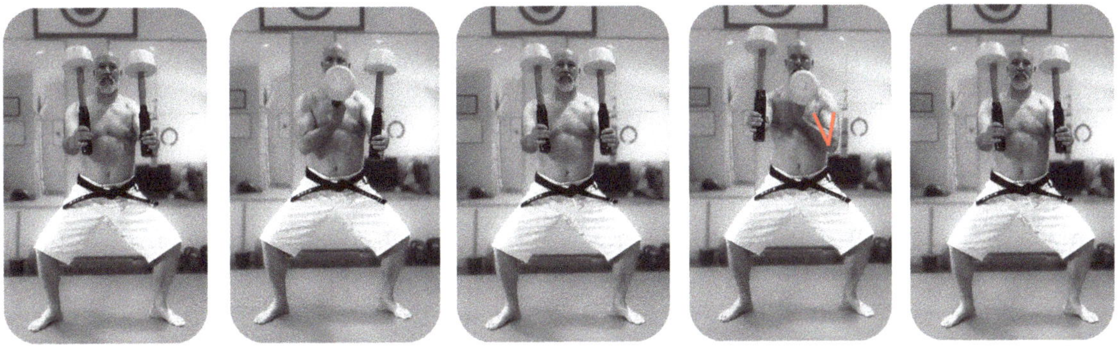

Center

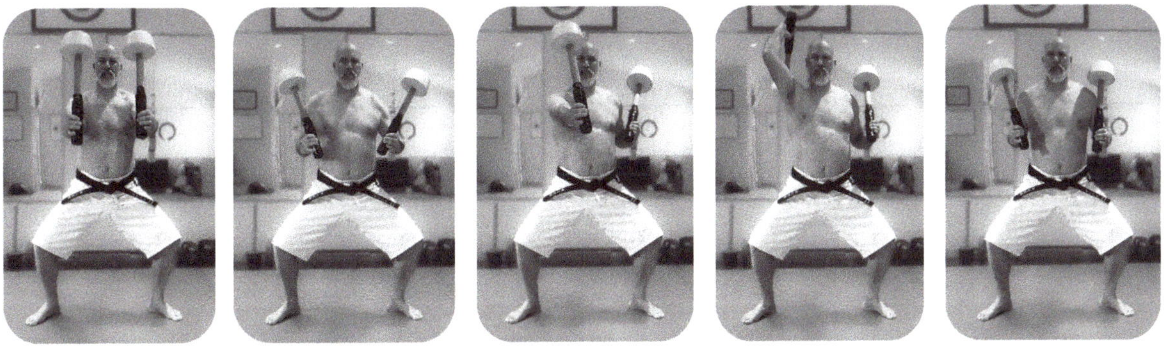

Out and over shoulder

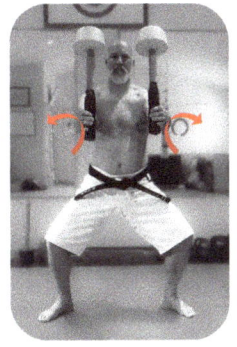
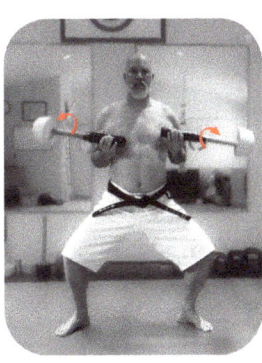
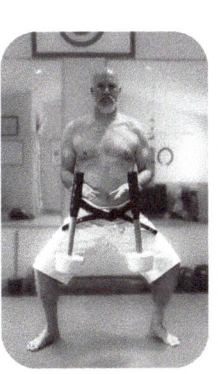
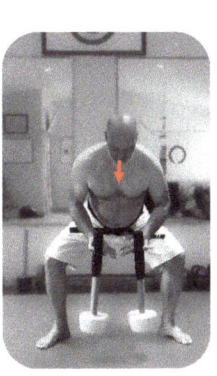

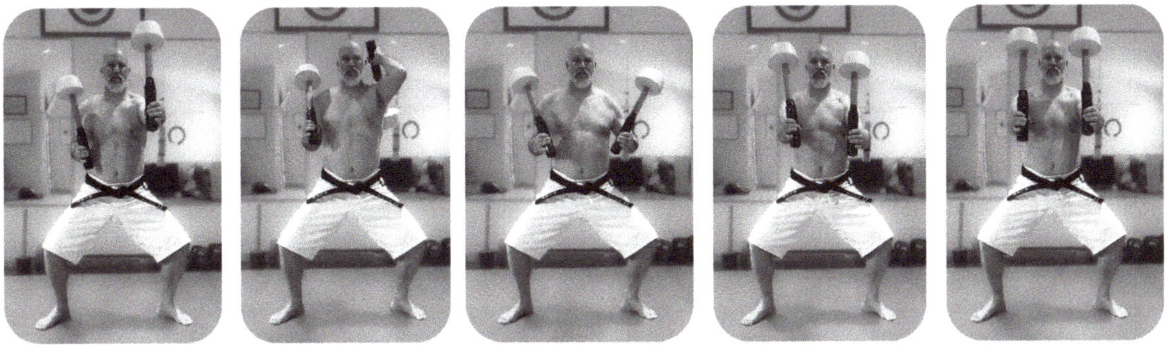

Reset

Kigu Undō

Preparation

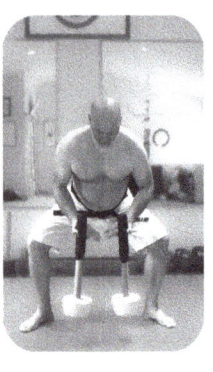
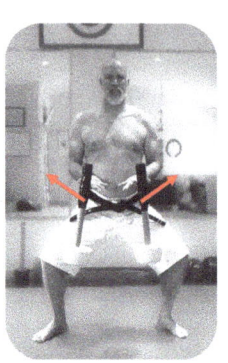

Weight position

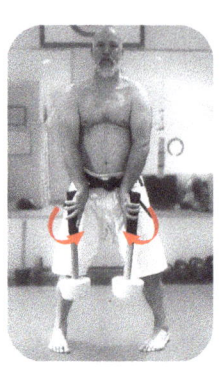
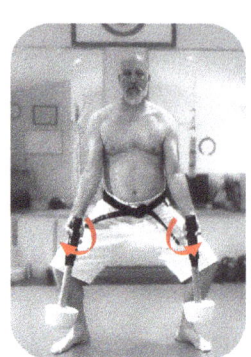

Zenkutsu

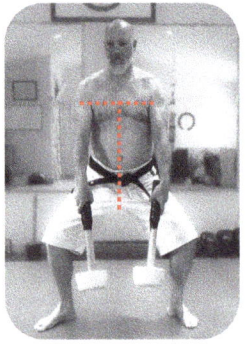
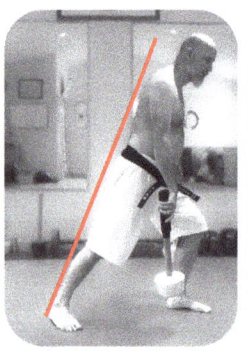
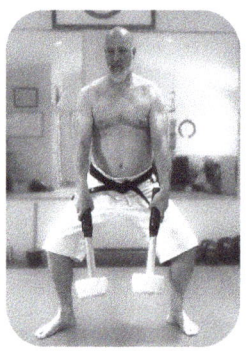
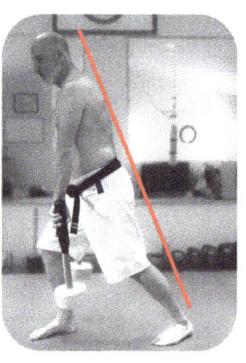

Maintain a straight line from the head to the back heel.

Neko Ashi

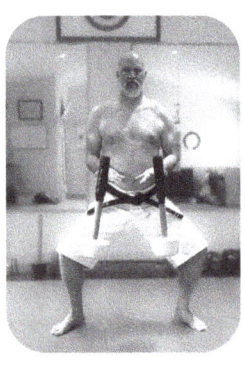
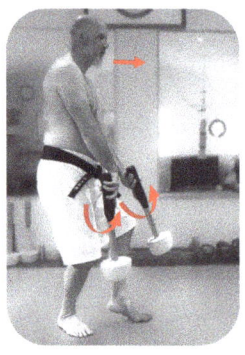
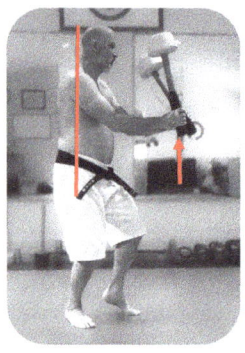
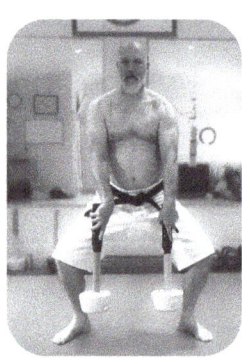
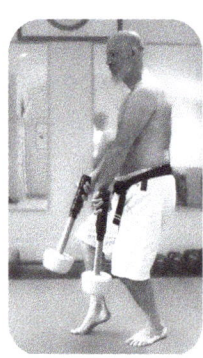

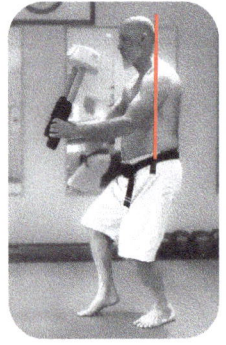
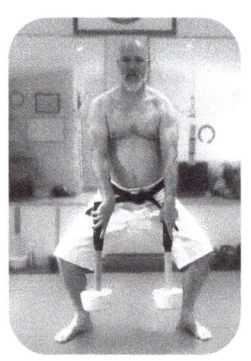

Body alignment is key and as important as strength building.

器具運動　　　　　　　　　　　Kigu Undō

Me, Soku, Te is not only when doing Kata; it is equally important throughout your training.

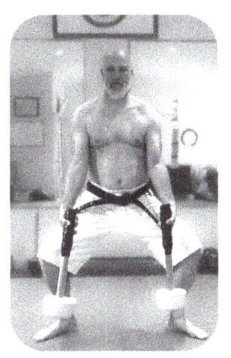 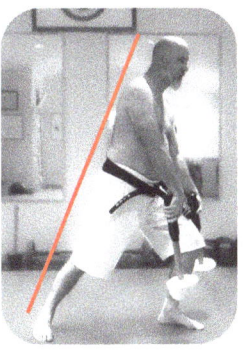 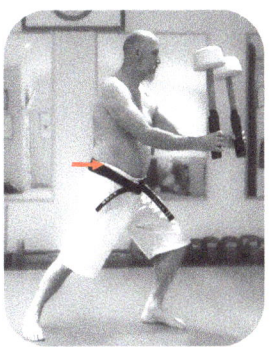 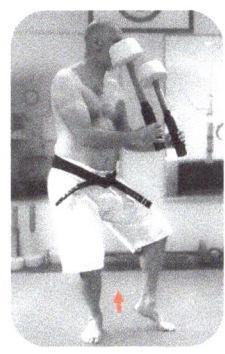

Turn, lean, pull back

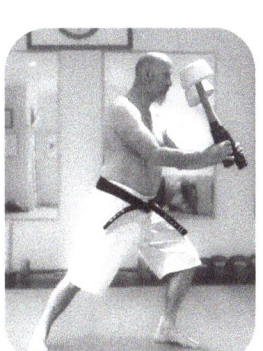 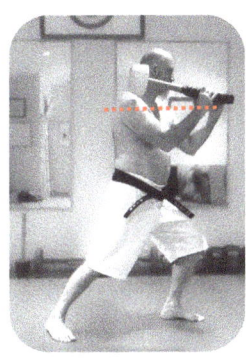 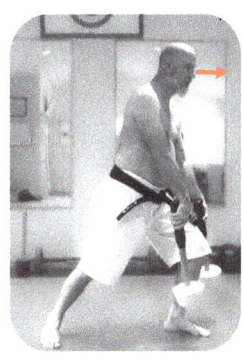 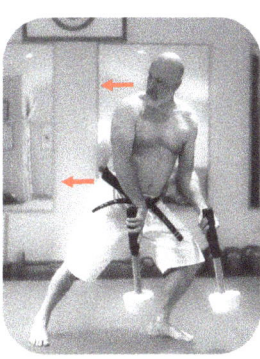

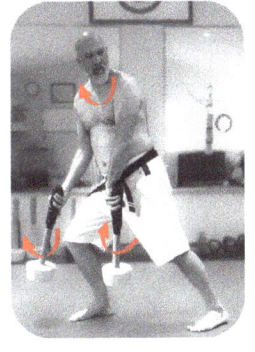 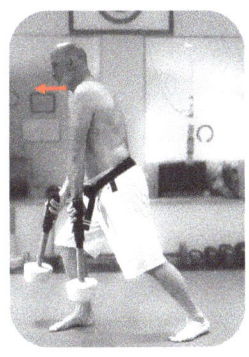 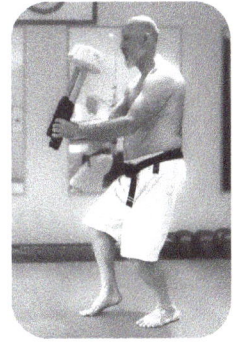 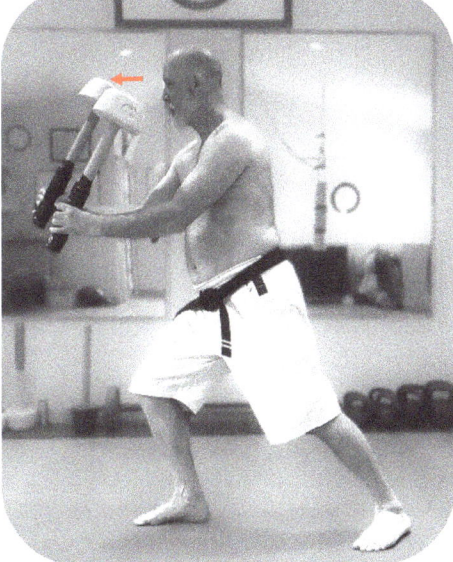

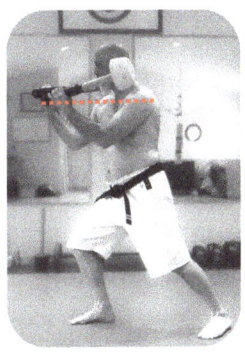 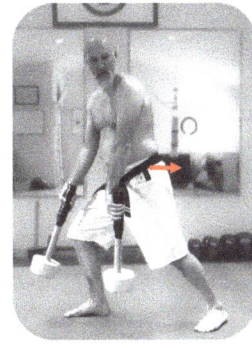 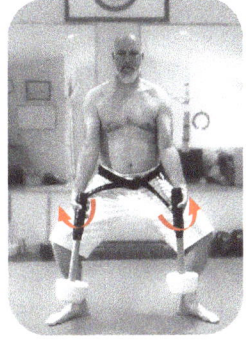

器具運動 Kigu Undō

Wrist hooks

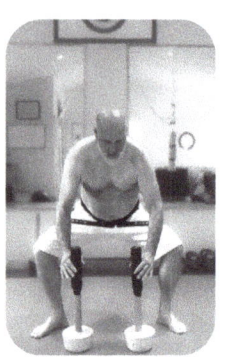 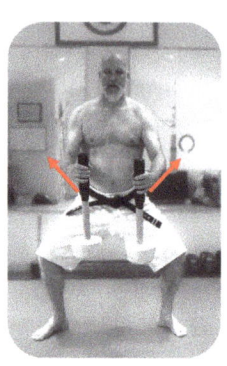 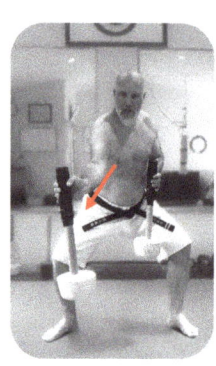 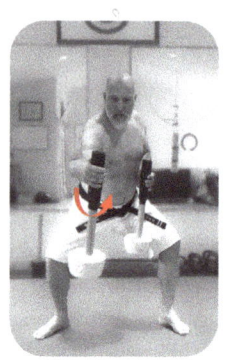

Note the reverse grip when lifting the Chiishi.

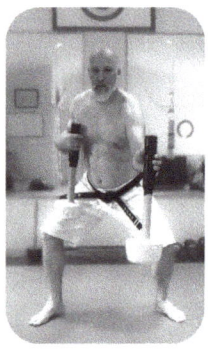 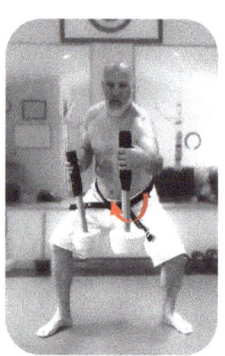 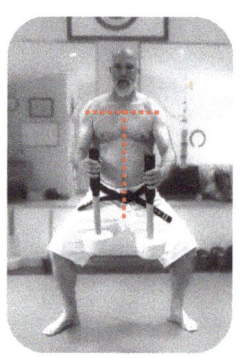 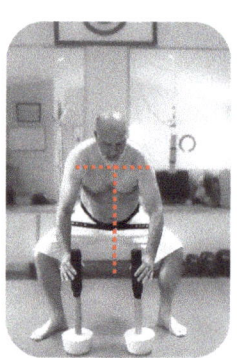

The palm pushes forward and then the wrist hooks to pull back.

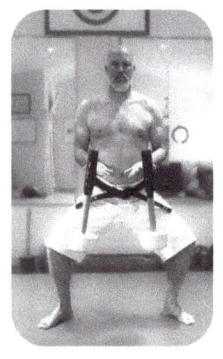 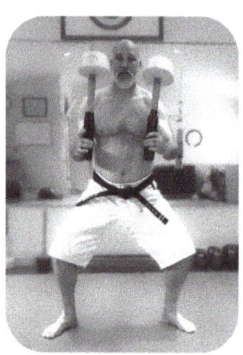 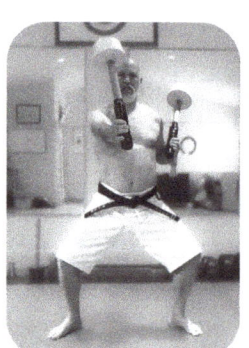 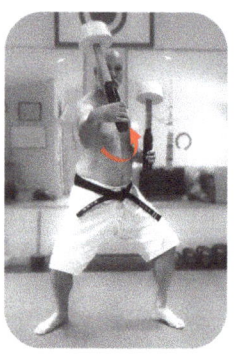

Push, hook, pull are done at each level; Jodan, Chudan, Gedan.

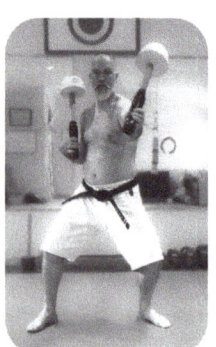 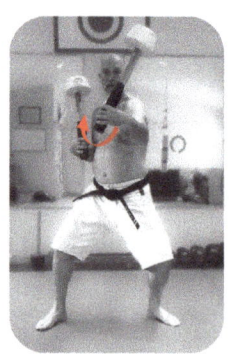 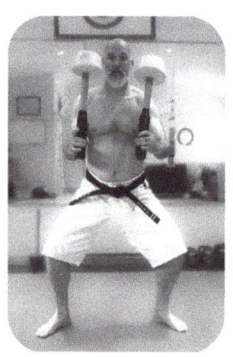 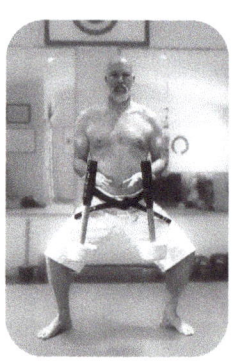

器具運動 Kigu Undō

Tan

Similar to the Chiishi exercise, the palm pushes forward and then the wrist hooks to pull back.

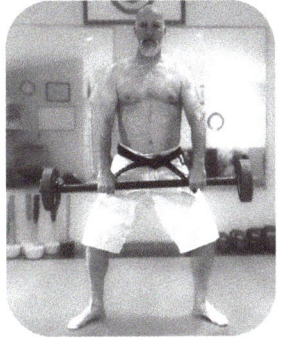
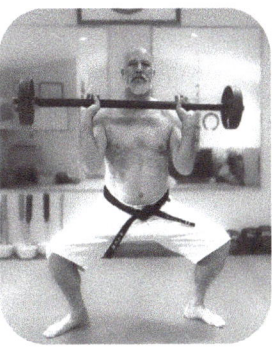
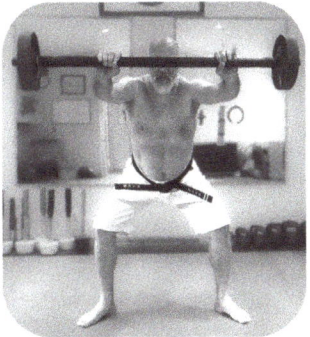
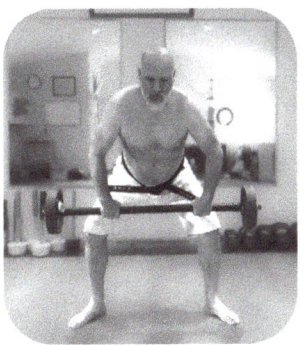

Forward reach

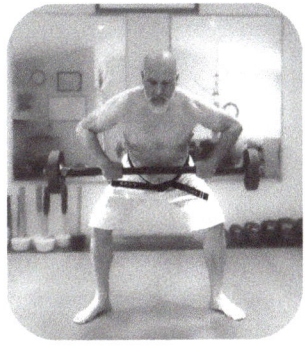
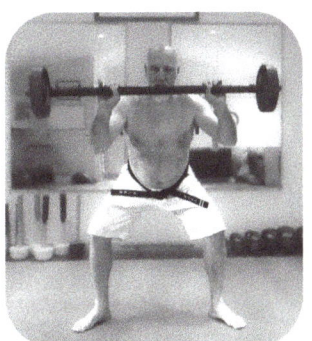
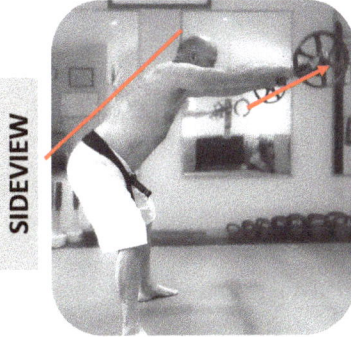
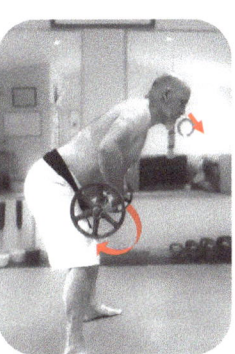

SIDEVIEW

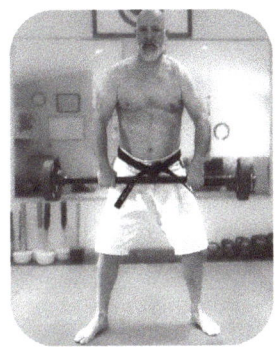
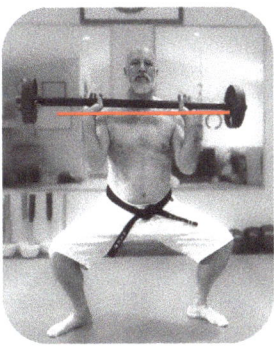
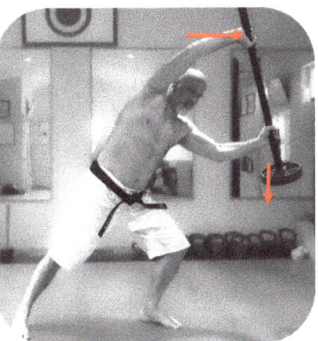
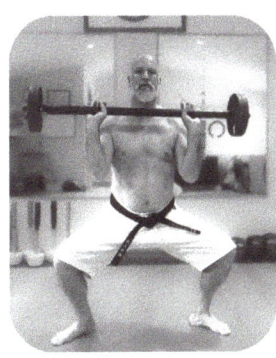

Lateral reach

Lower the bottom wheel of the Tan as much as possible, while maintaining proper form with the torso.

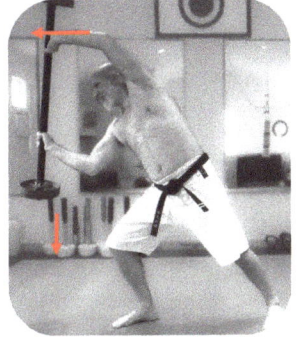
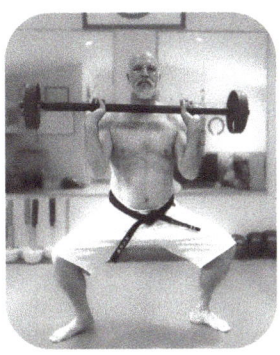
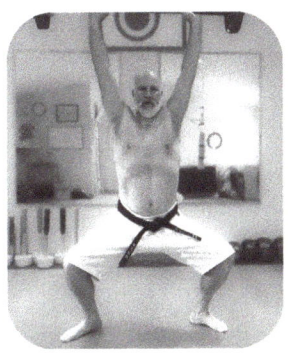
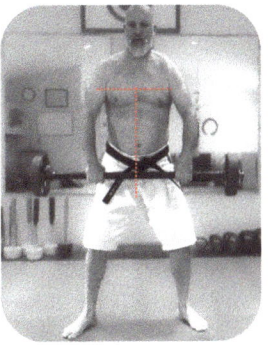

Kigu Undō

器具運動

Kami

Torso twist

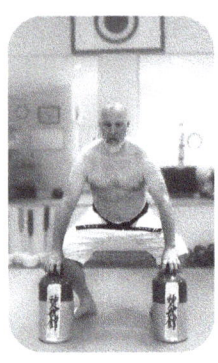
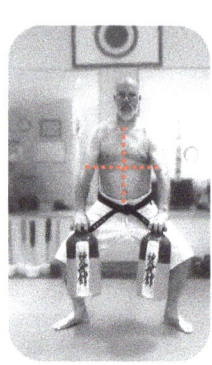
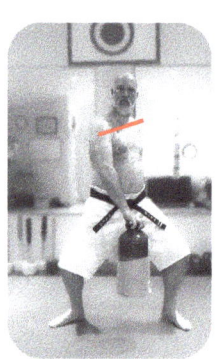
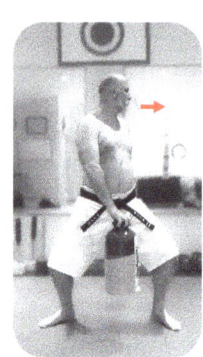

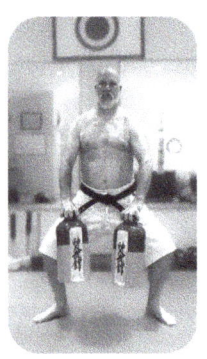
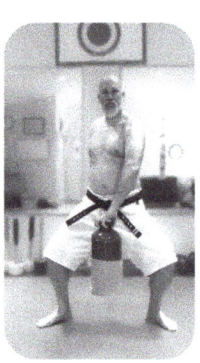
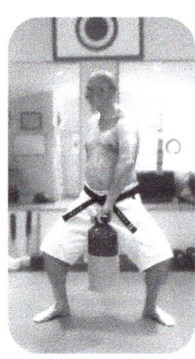
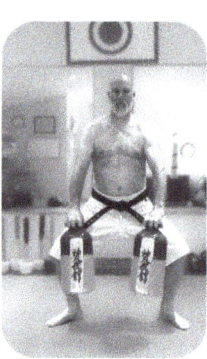

Most of the same principles discussed for Chiishi apply to Kami as well. Key things to consider are selecting the appropriate weight, how to pick up the Kami from the ground, correct posture, balance, Chinkuchi, and focus on Me, Soku, Te.

Neko Ashi

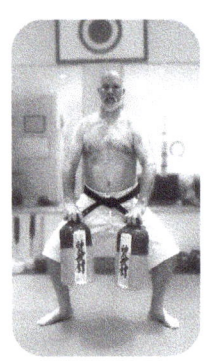
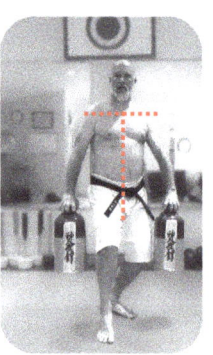
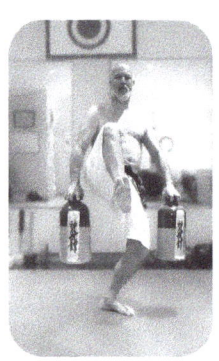
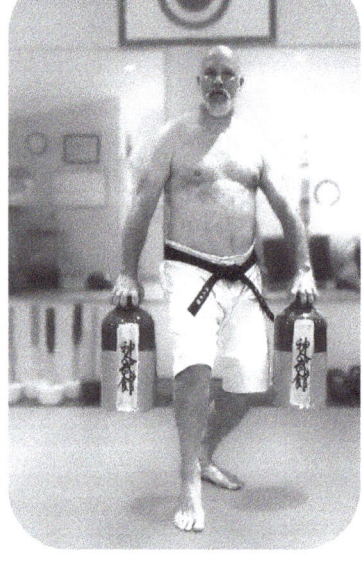

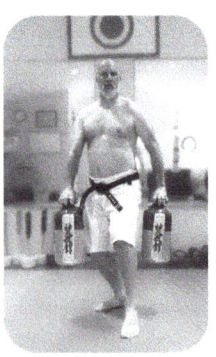
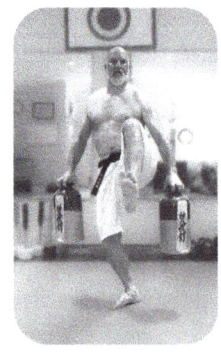
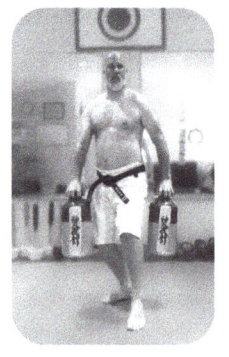

70

器具運動　　Kigu Undō

Stepping

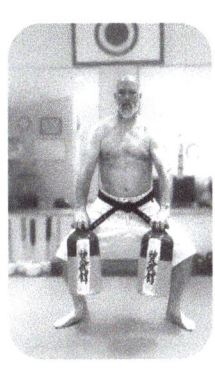 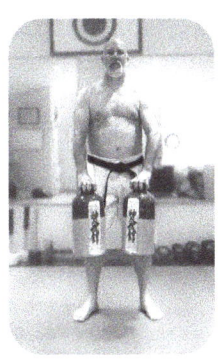 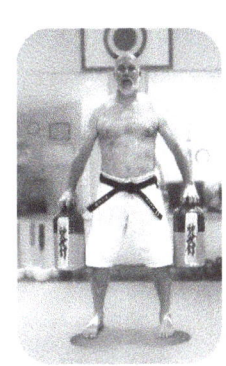 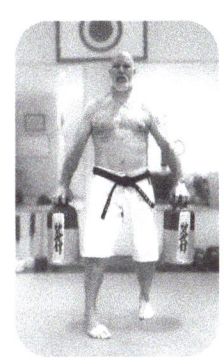 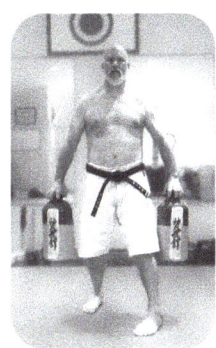

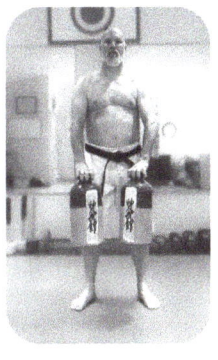 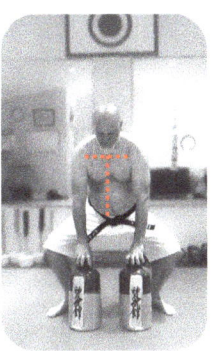 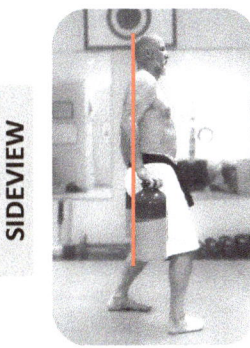

SIDEVIEW

The one key difference with Kami is the grip. Ensure that jars have a lip that allows for proper thumb and finger position. The mouth of the jar should fill the palm of the hand.

Arm extensions

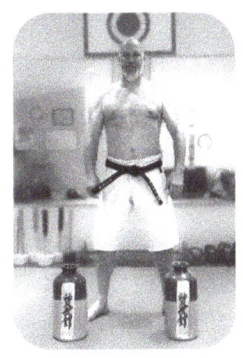 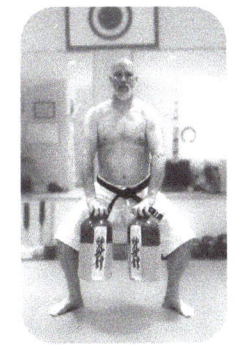 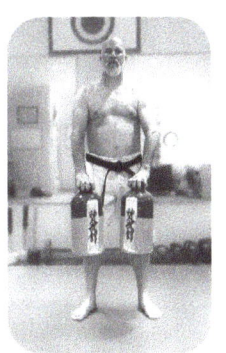

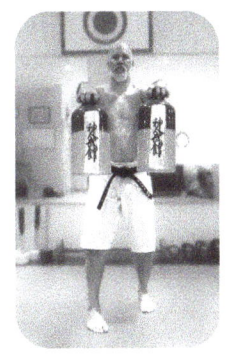 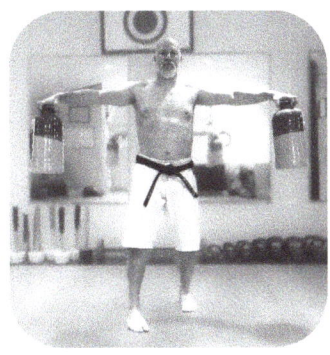 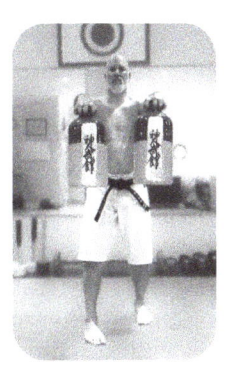

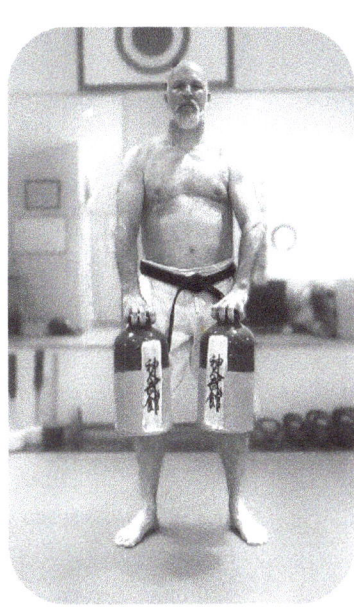

器具運動 Kigu Undō

Arm extensions

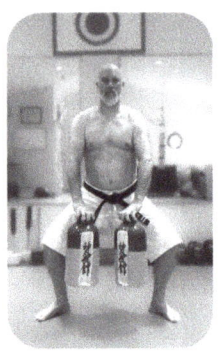 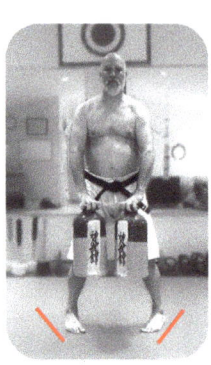 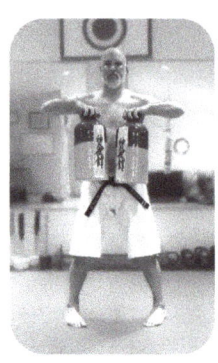 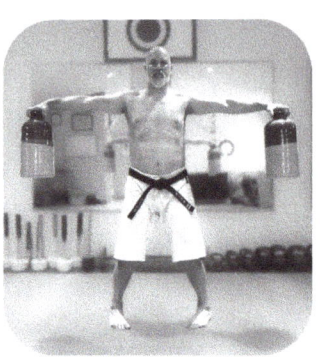 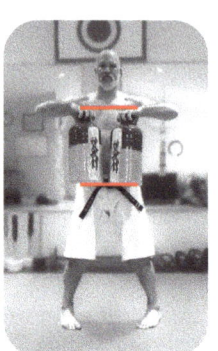

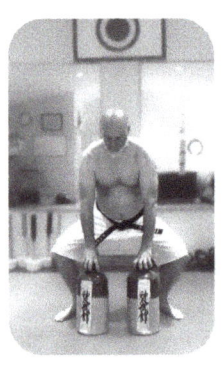 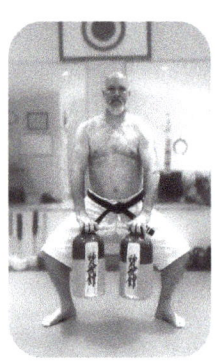 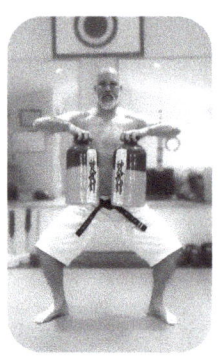 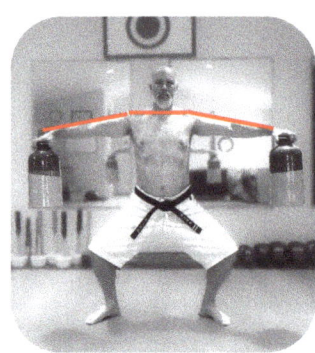 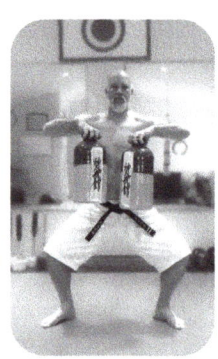

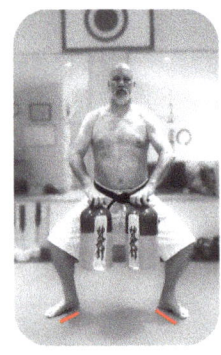 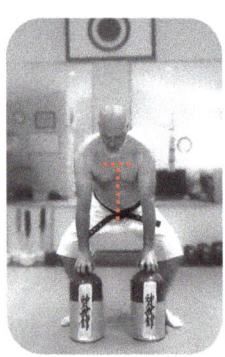

When opening the arms, keep the height just below the shoulders, at a slight downward angle similar to executing Miji Nagashi Jichi.

器具運動 — Kigu Undō

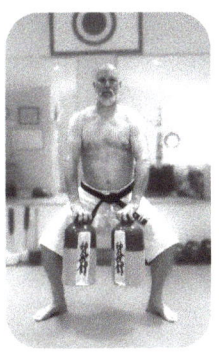 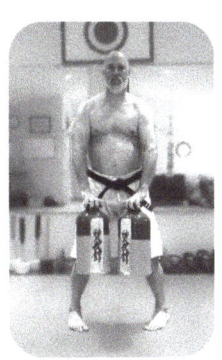 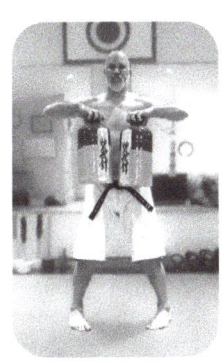 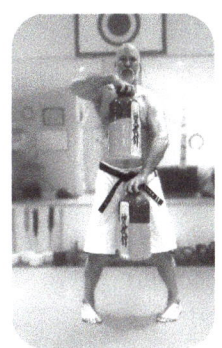 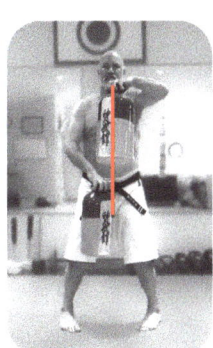

Front rolls

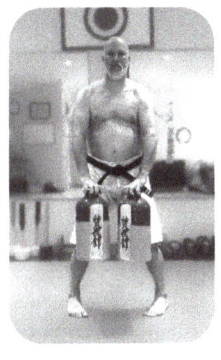 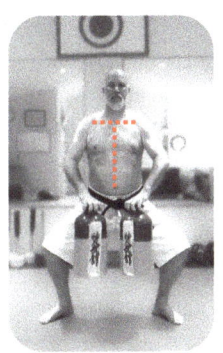 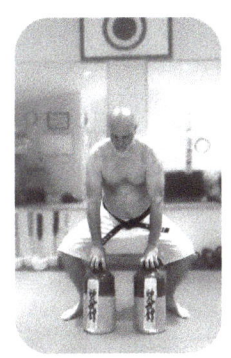

Kami training is typically done in Shiko Dachi, Shizentai, Naihanchi Dachi, and Neko Ashi Dachi.

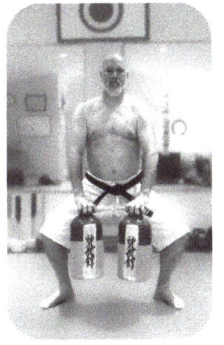 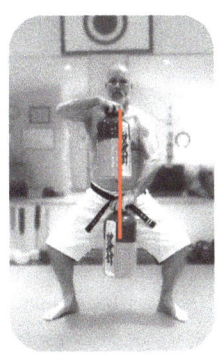 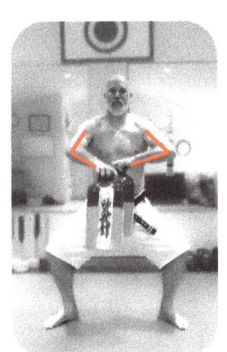

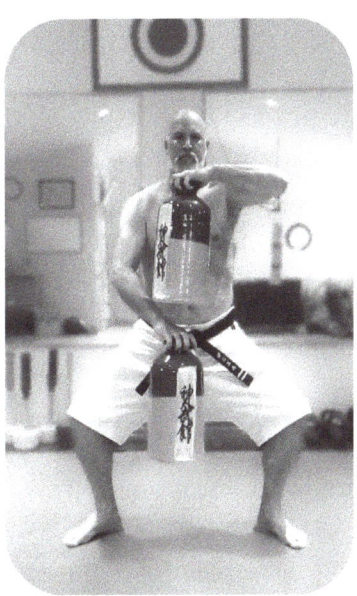

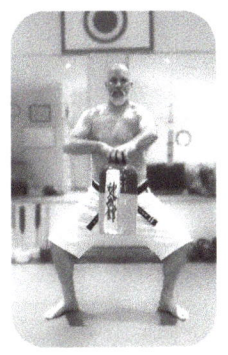 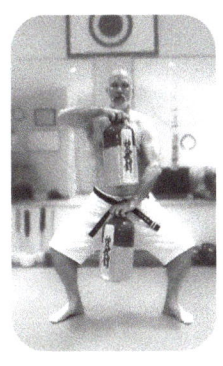 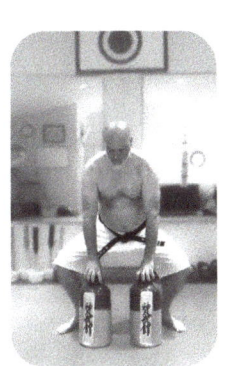

When the jars are in front of the body, move both in a forward circle and a reverse circle motion.

73

器具運動　　　　　　　　　　　　　　　　Kigu Undō

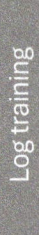
Log training

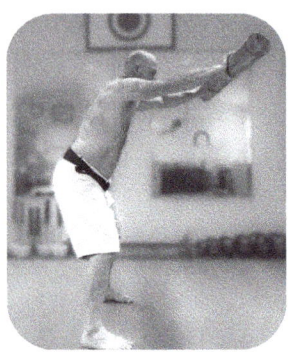 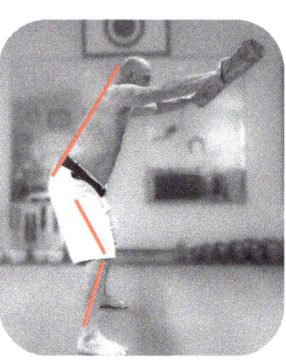 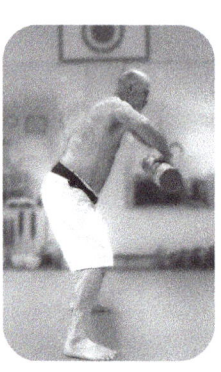 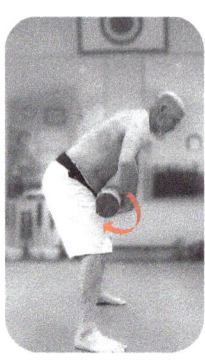 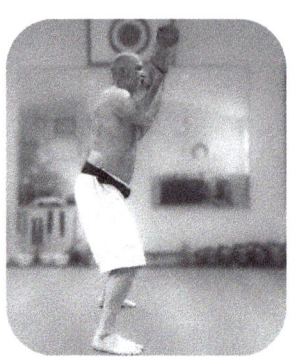

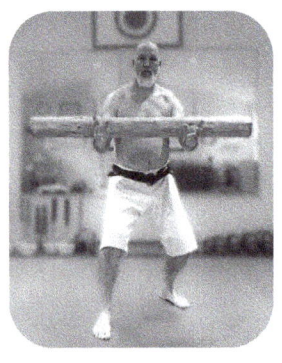 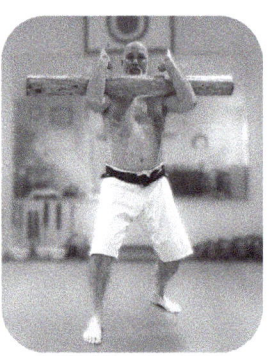 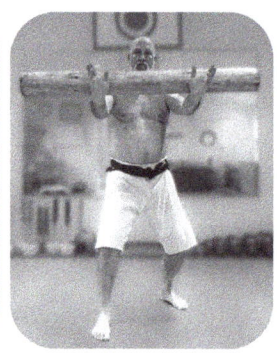 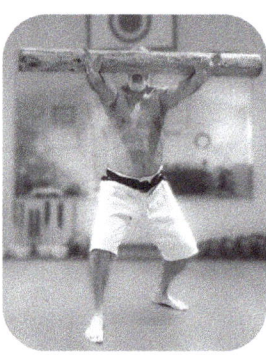 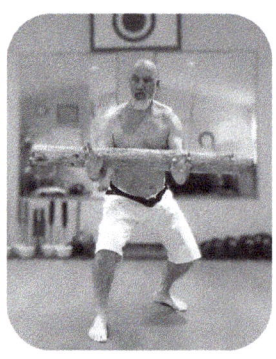

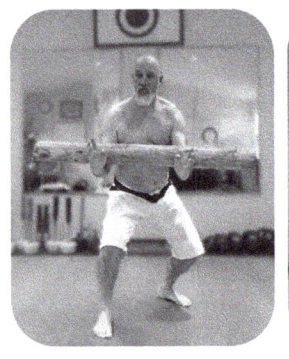 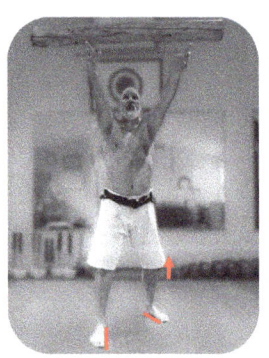 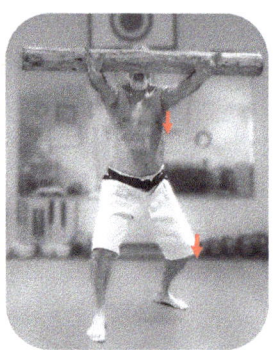 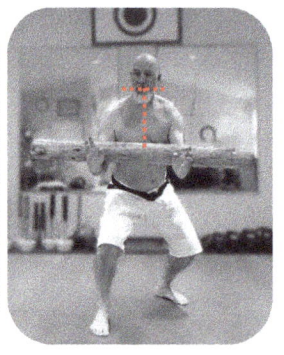

If the log is small enough to grip, then all the exercises for Tan are also applicable to the log.

SIDEVIEW

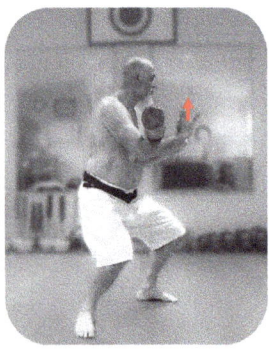 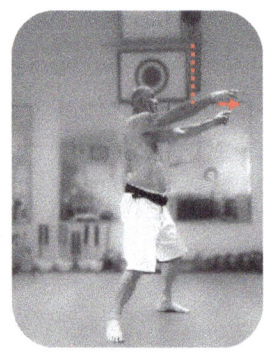 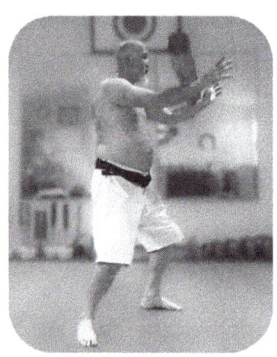 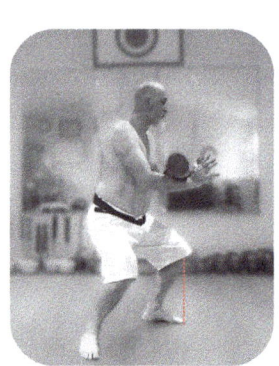

器具運動 Kigu Undō

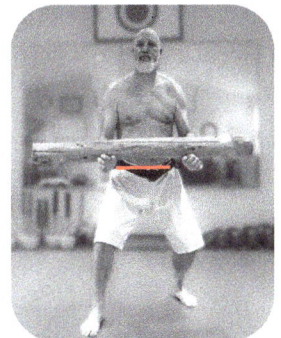 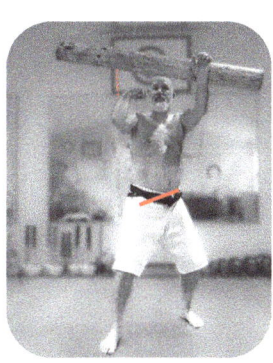 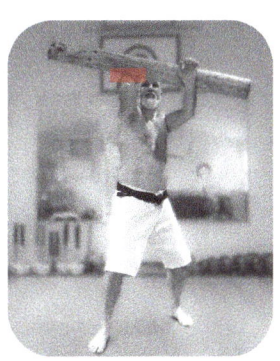 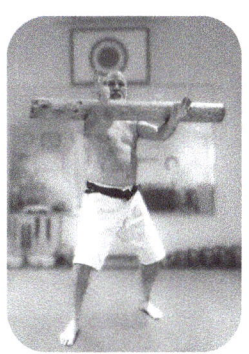 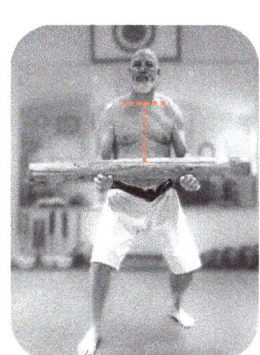

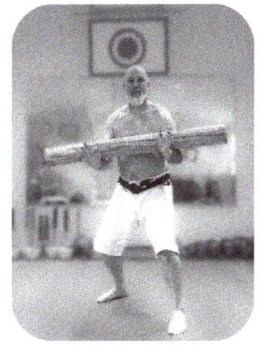 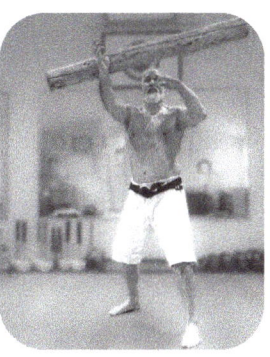 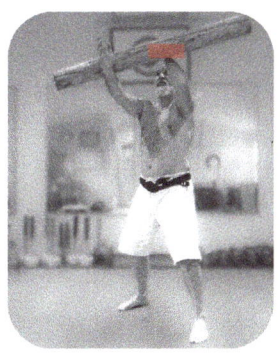 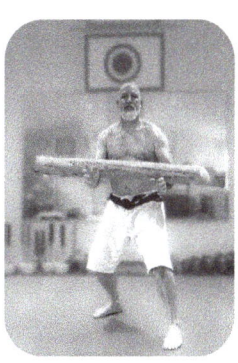

Block the log with one arm using Age Uke, and return the arm below the log to hold it on the way down.

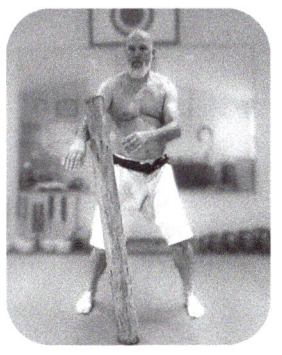 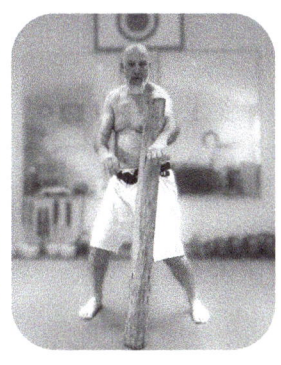 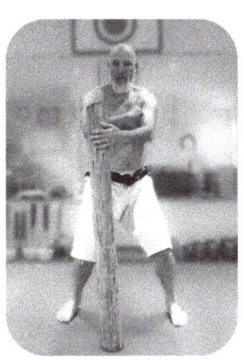 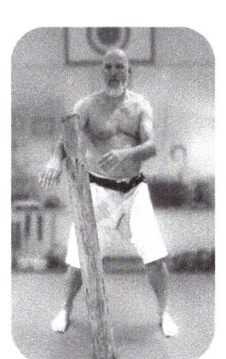 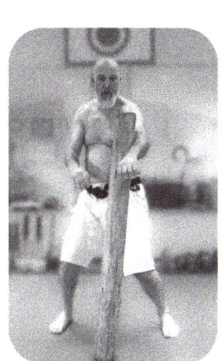

Standing log

A standing log is a good substitute for a Sagi Machiwara.

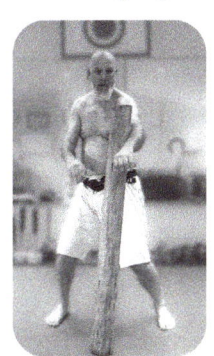 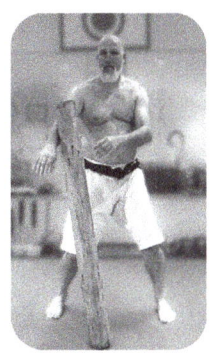 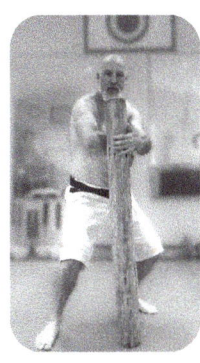 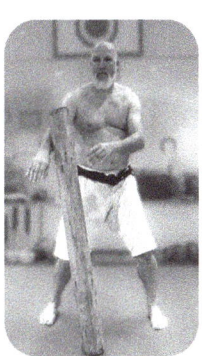 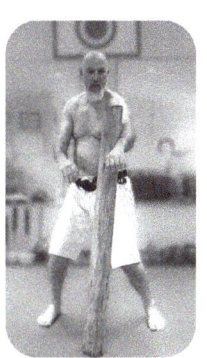 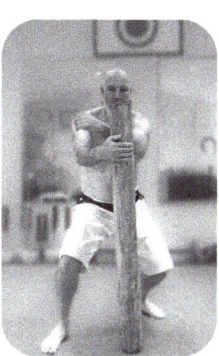

器具運動 Kigu Undō

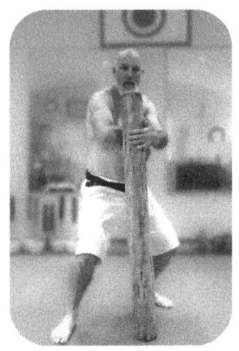
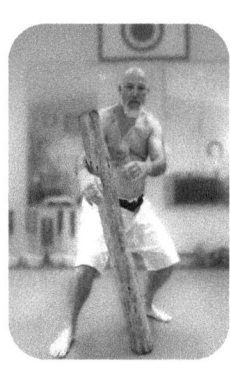
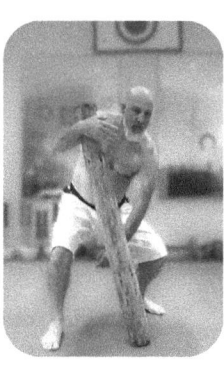
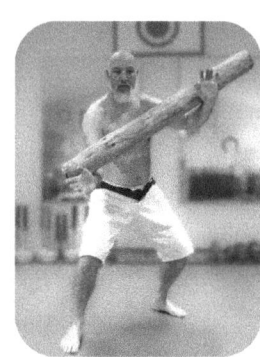
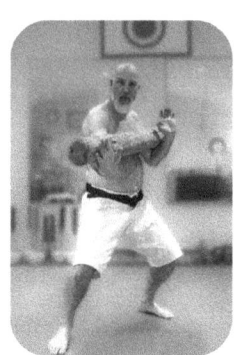

Leg hooks, sweeps, and lifting of an opponent can be done either with a partner or a log.

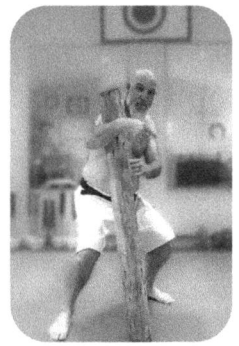
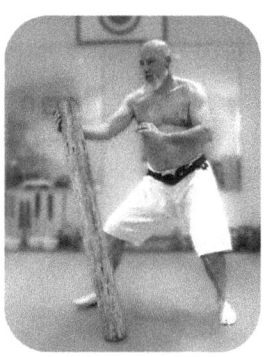
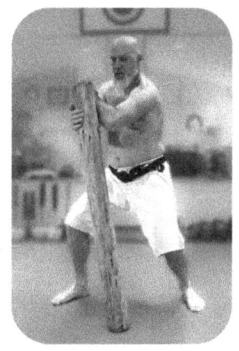
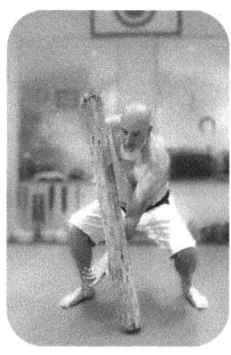
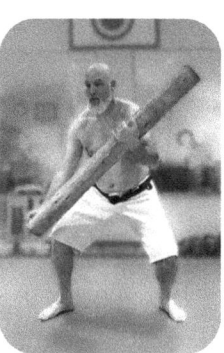

Training with a log is an a easy substitute for a Tan, Sagi Machiwara, or a partner, and is best done outside, since training in the Dojo will add serious consequences when a mistake is made. Just like when we say, the Machiwara is your teacher and will make you aware when you make a mistake, this holds true for training with a log indoors.

器具運動   Kigu Undō

Below are just a few examples of the different exercises that exist with these very simple and easy to use tools.

Pull back and grip with the toes when rolling forward; keep the toes up as in Tenshin or Kata.

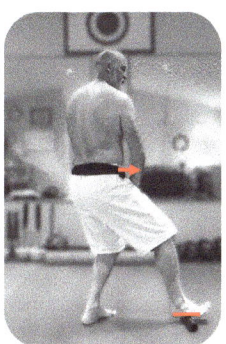 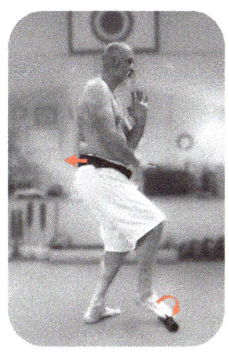 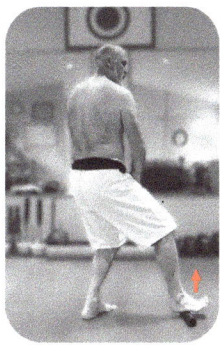 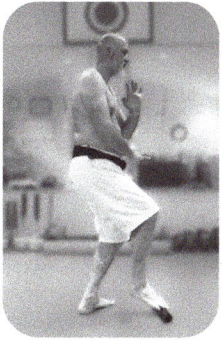

Foot roller

Start fighting distance away, kick with either leg at speed between the uprights. Traditionally done with Shoji screens slightly ajar.

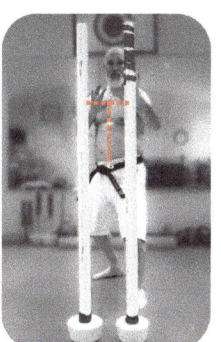 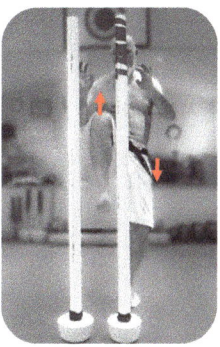 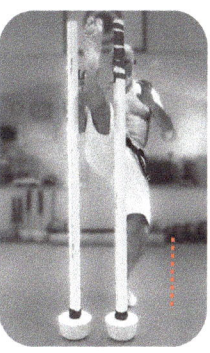 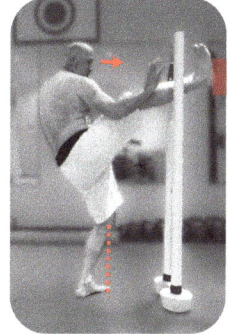

SIDEVIEW

Uprights

Working the hand and grip position while doing Kata or other solo practice.

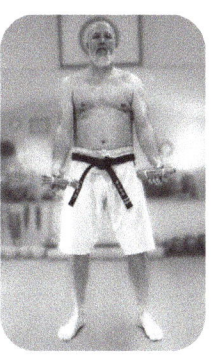 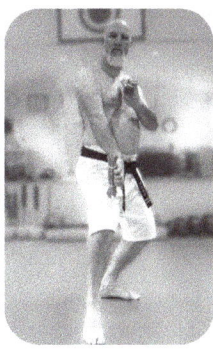 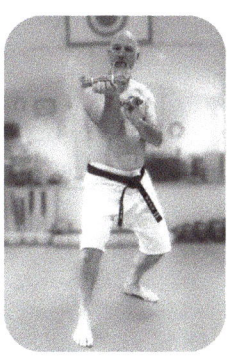 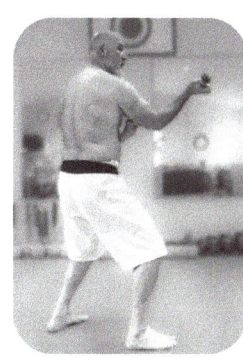

SIDEVIEW

Nigiri Dama

器具運動 Kigu Undō

Short stick

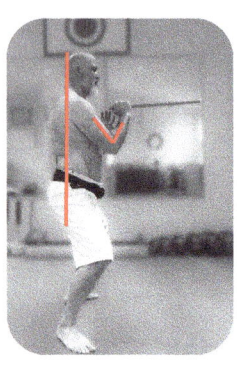 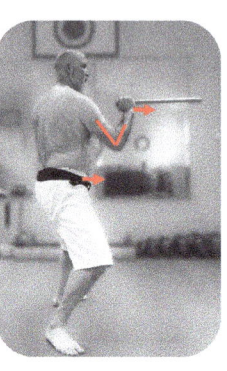 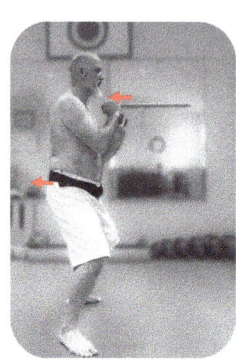

Do not stretch or reach with the arm. Use the hips to make the forward motion.

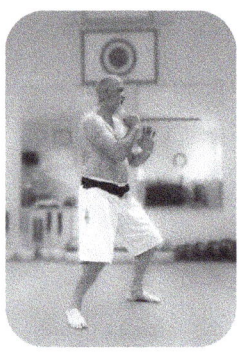 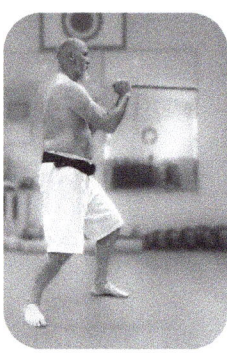 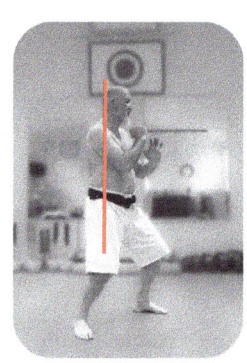

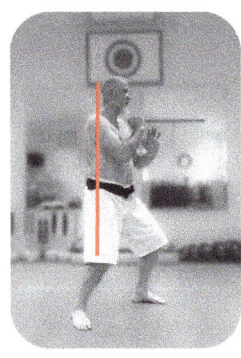 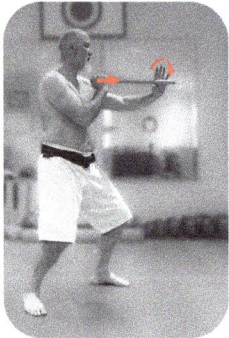 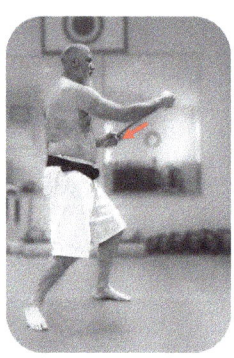 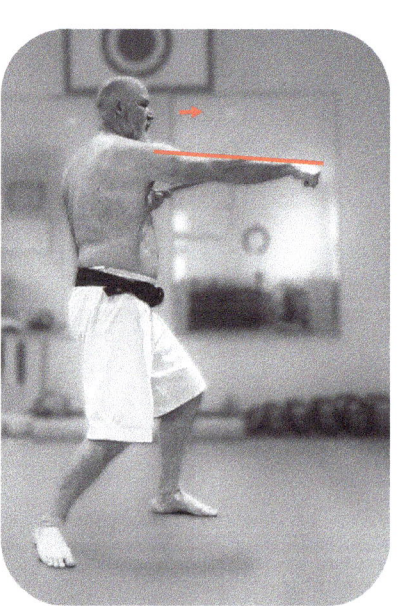

The striking arm should follow the line of the stick. Practice both as Kukan Tsuki as well as with Machiwara.

器具運動 Kigu Undō

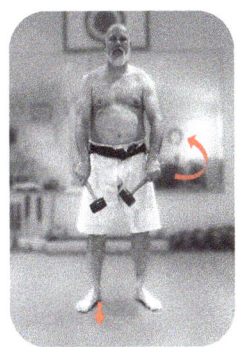 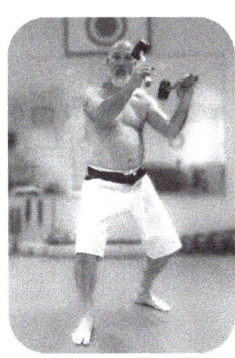 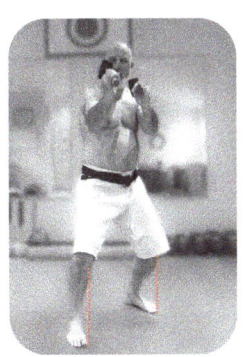

Hammers, similar to Nigiri Dama can, and should, be used for both free solo practice as well as while doing Kata.

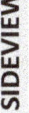 SIDEVIEW

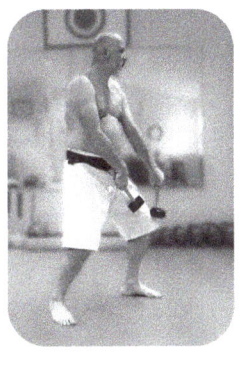 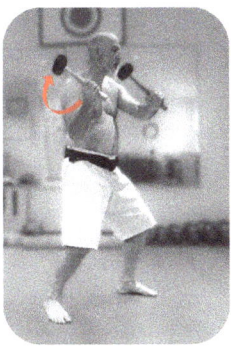 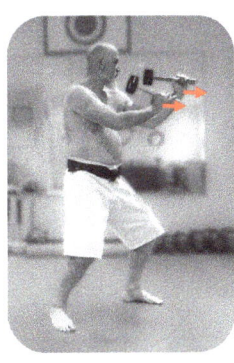 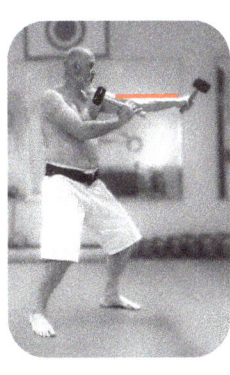 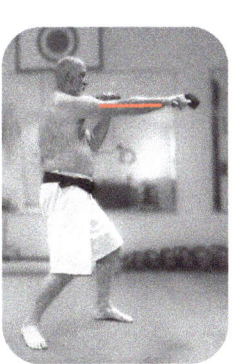

器具運動   Kigu Undō

Nunchaku

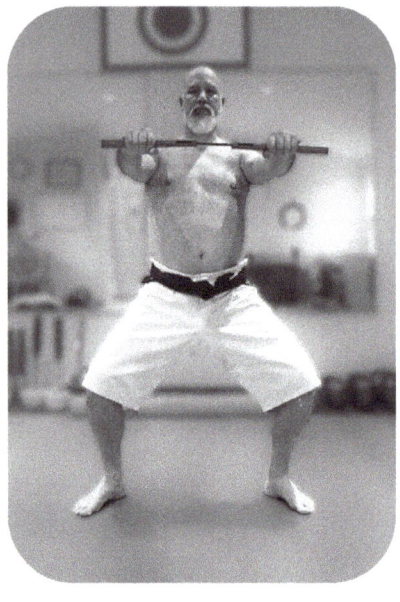

Kokyu, breathing exercises. Done in Shiko Dachi, using slow and forced breath (Go).

External rotation.

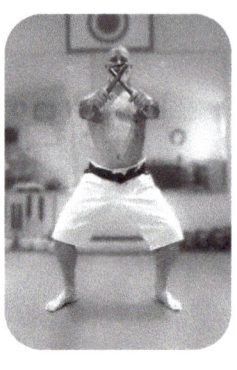 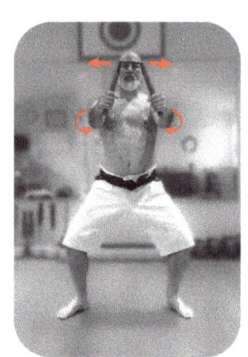

Internal rotation.

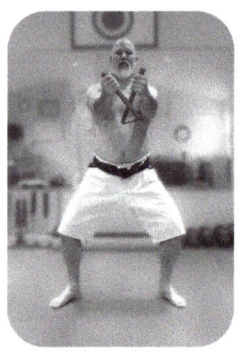 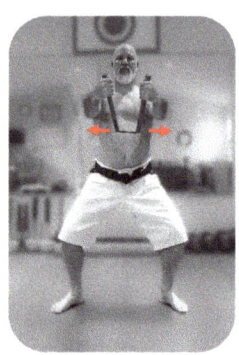

Pull / Push combination.

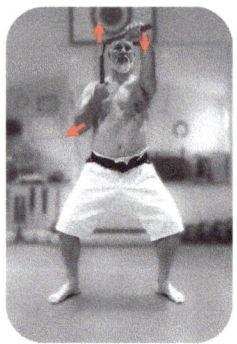 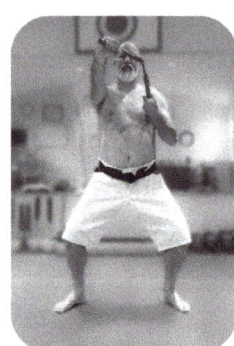

Each of the 3 exercises is done at each of the 3 height levels.

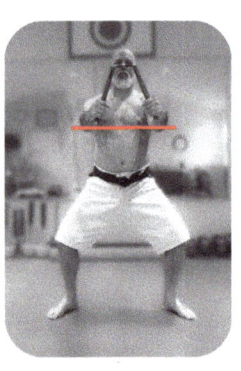 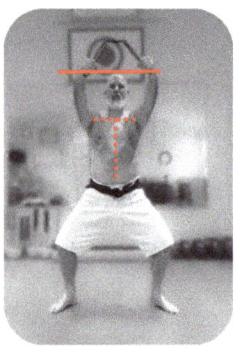 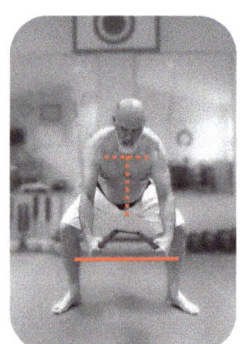

SIDEVIEW

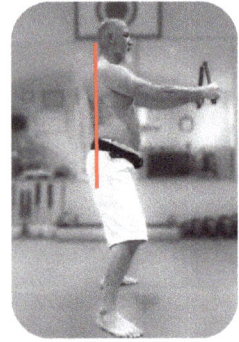 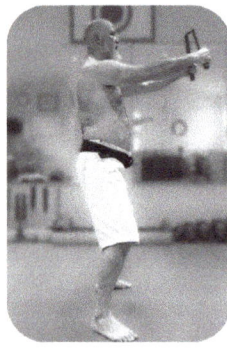 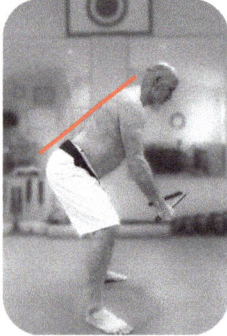

Although this exercise is done with Nunchaku, Kobudo was never taught at the Onaga Dojo. The Nunchaku are a training tool like the rest.

器具運動 — Kigu Undō

Cutting paper is a very effective way to learn and practice speed and focus. It's important to practice all 5 basic Tsuki.

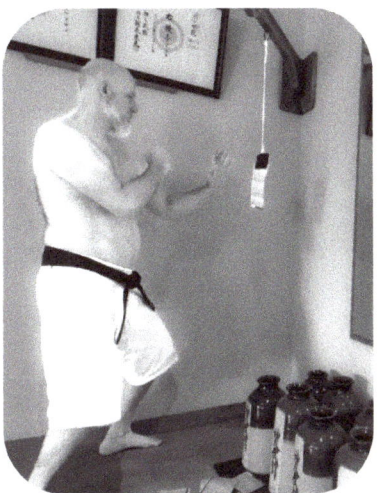
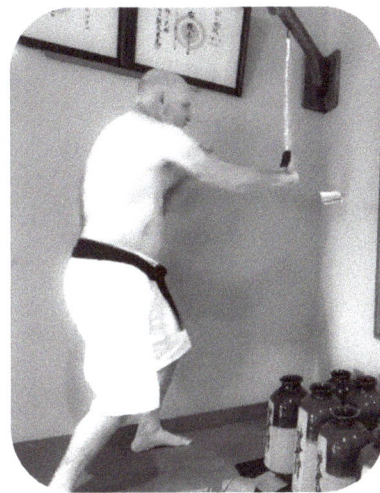
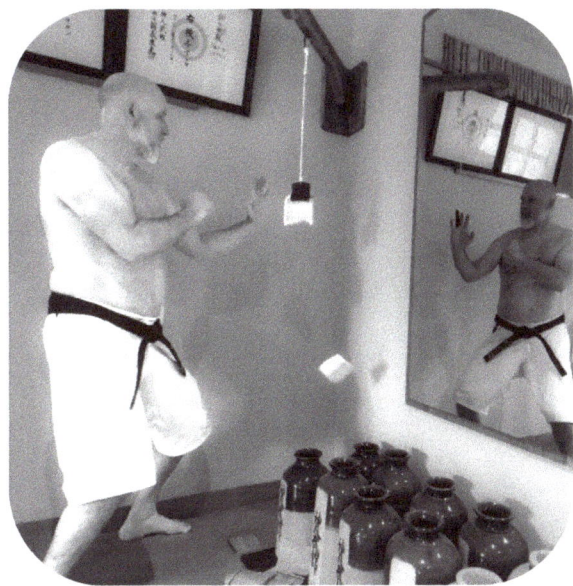

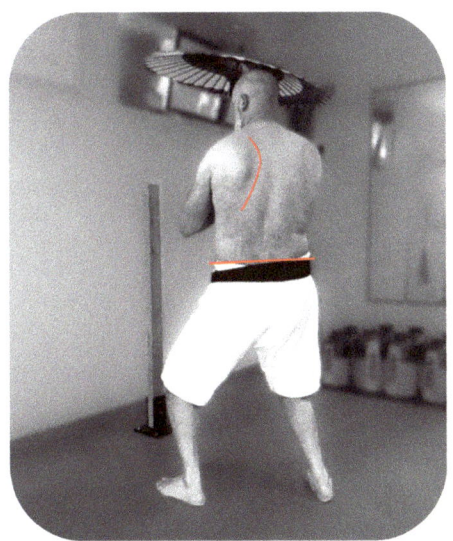
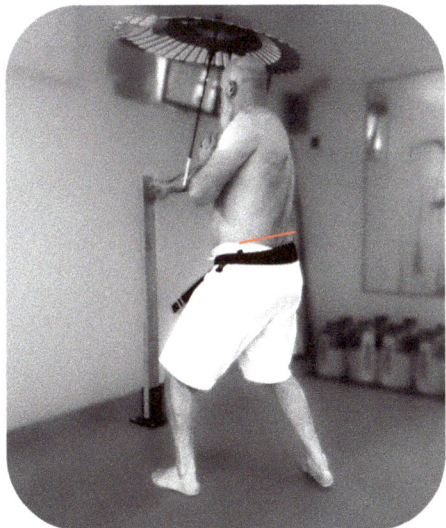

A less common, but very effective, way to practice speed is by holding a paper umbrella in the striking hand. Release, strike the Machiwara, and catch the umbrella in a single smooth motion.

Fully extended Tsuki, retractor to the center of the chest, hips square when striking.

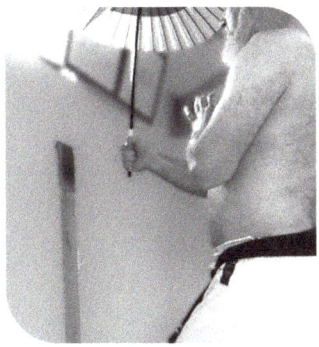
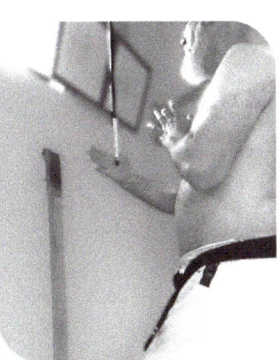
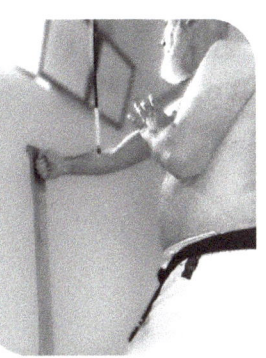
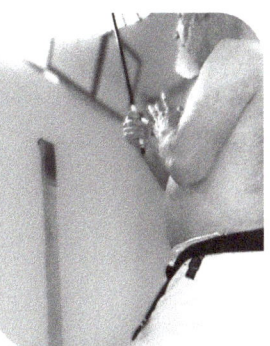

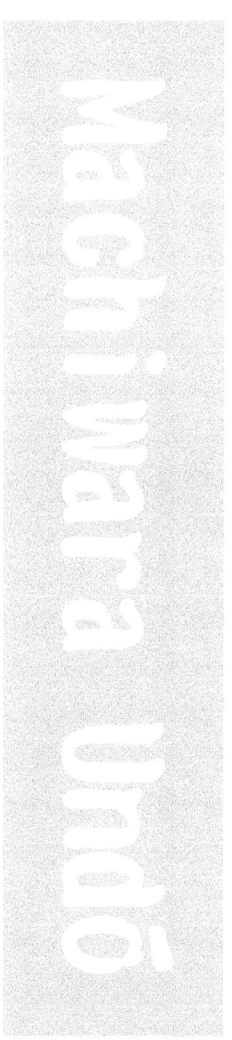

Machiwara Undō

Machiwara, the Okinawan pronunciation of the Japanese Makiwara (巻藁), which literally means wrapped straw, is used as the target in Japanese archery. Modern Karate Machiwara are rarely made with straw, but the name is still used and has morphed into meaning something like "striking tool." There are three types of Machiwara in our Dojo: Tachi Machiwara, or standing Machiwara, referring to it being fixed to the ground (sometimes a wall); Sagi Machiwara, literally a "hanging Machiwara"; and Ti Machiwara, meaning "hand" Machiwara, which is a small block held in the hand as a striking surface.

The construction techniques for making each of these different types of Machiwara are critical for their effectiveness as a training tool. The height, weight, shape, angle, and density are all considerations when building Machiwara.

マチワラ運動　　　　　　　　　　　Machiwara Undō

Proper distance, both for Heisoku Dachi as well as in Jigotai, is to have the Machiwara at the middle knuckles.

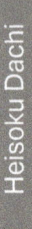 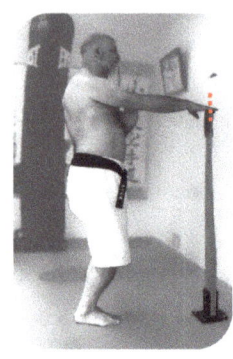 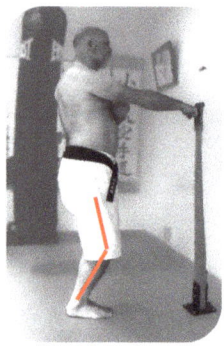 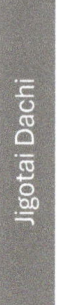 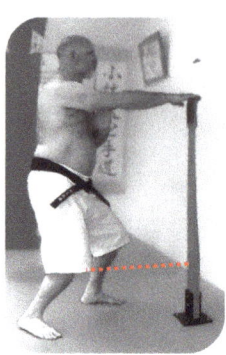 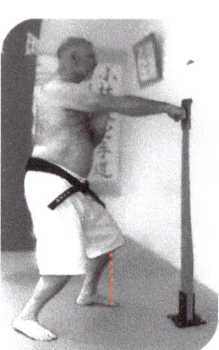

Look prior to Hikite and again before striking.   The strike travels down towards the heels; let it push you back.

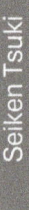 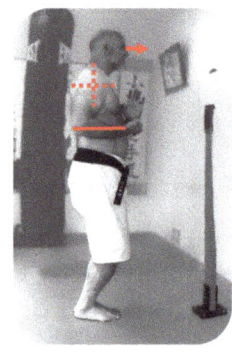 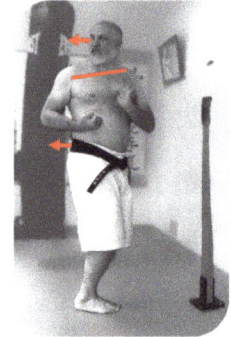 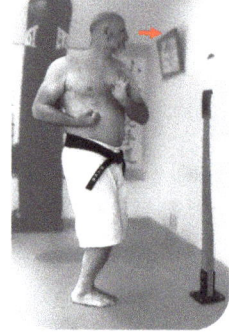 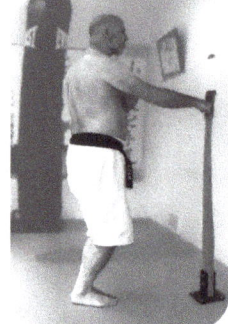 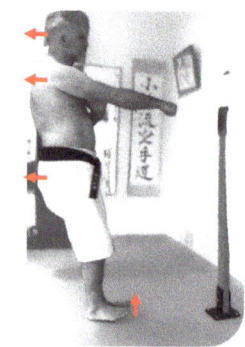

Straight mid-level strike.   From the outside striking in.

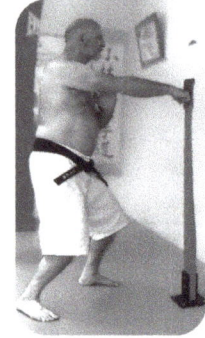 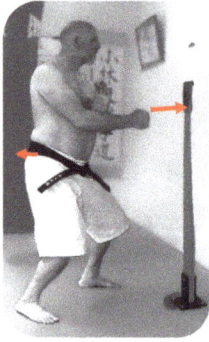 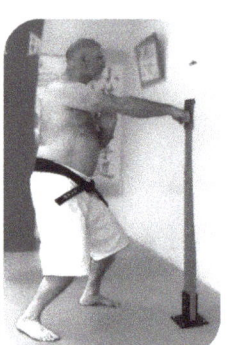 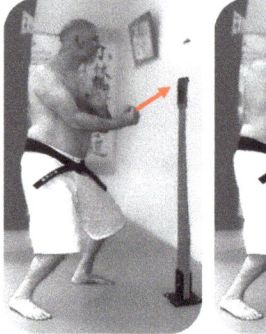 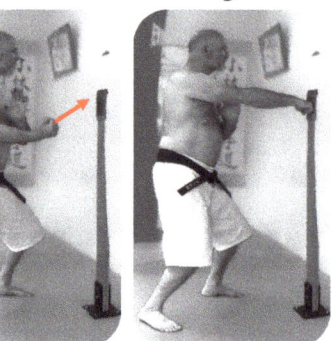

From the inside striking across.   From above downward.   From below rising.

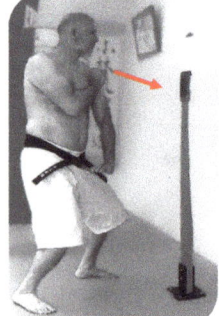 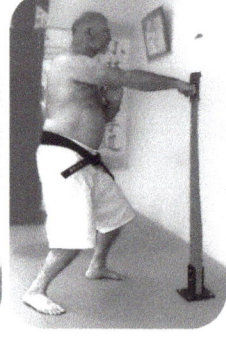 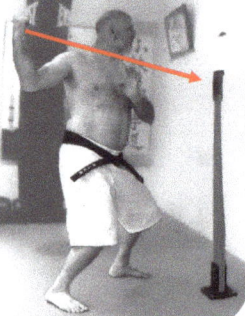 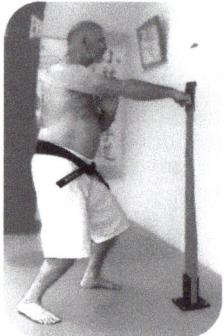 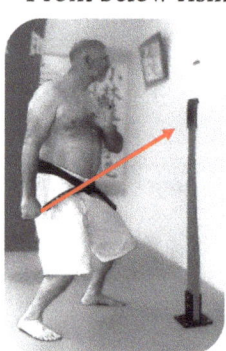 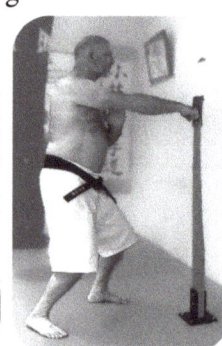

マチワラ運動 Machiwara Undō

The five basic strikes, each done with the other arm blocking. The blocking arm uses the striking arm in place of what would be the opponent's technique. After the block is executed, the arm is extracted in order to use it to strike, while keeping the pressing blocking (Osae Uke) or touching hand (Sawaru Te) in position.

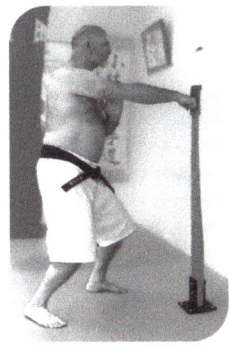 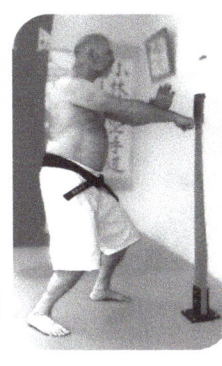 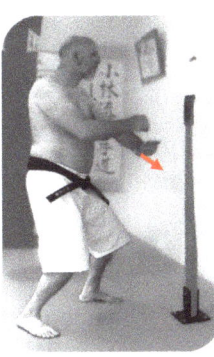 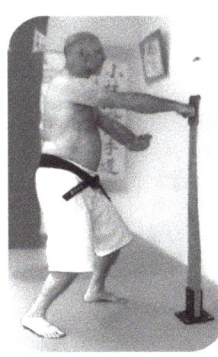

Downward Osae Uke and a straight mid-level strike.

Five directions two hands

Push across the body, strike in.

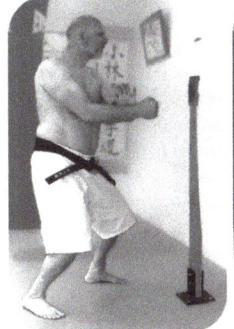 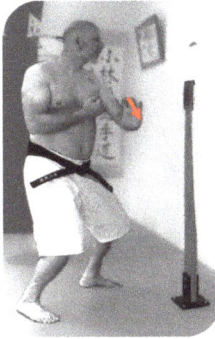 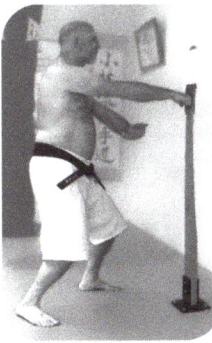

Hook out, strike across the body.

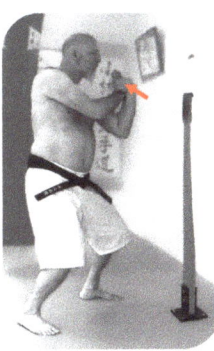 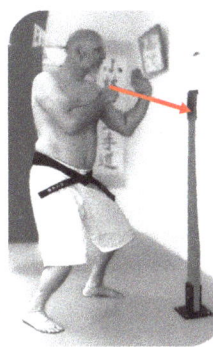 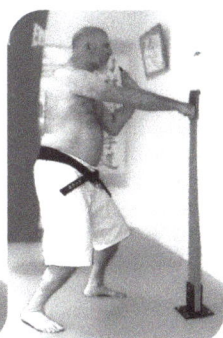

Rising block, downward strike.

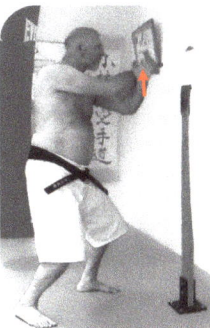 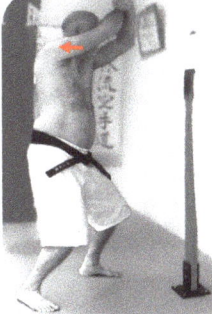 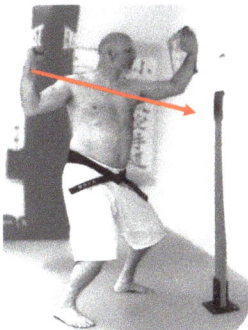

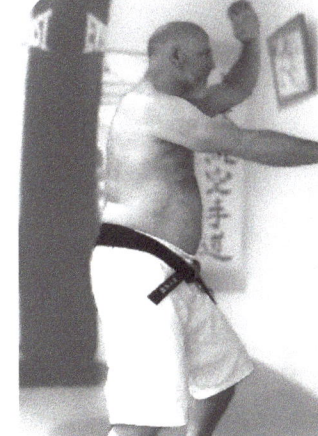

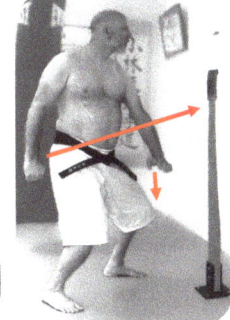 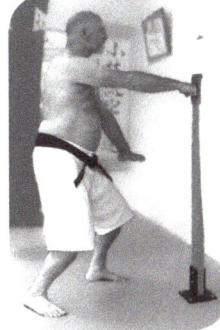

Downward block rising strike.

マチワラ運動　　　　　　　　Machiwara Undō

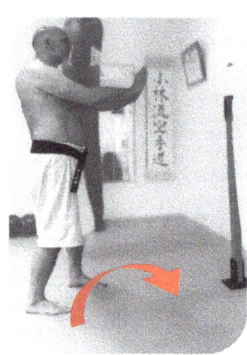 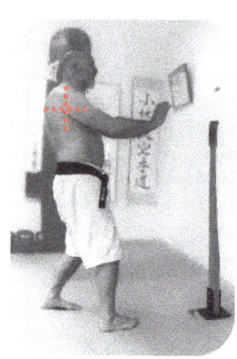 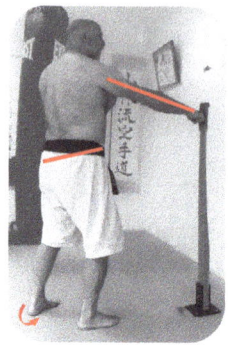 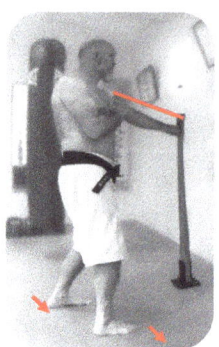 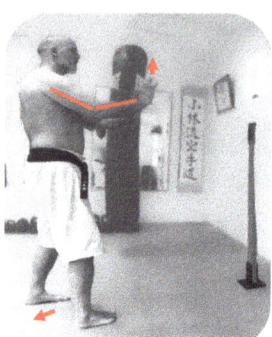

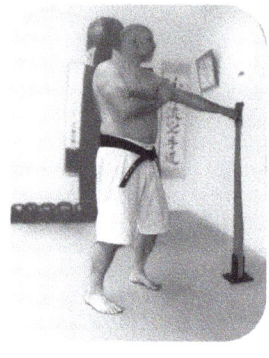 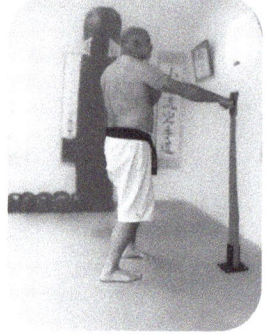 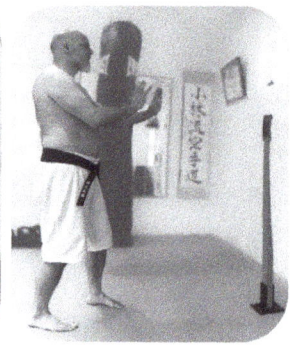

When stepping forward, focus on cranking the rear leg in order to have it thrust the striking hip forward, resulting in Oi Tsuki.

On the lateral shuffles, the feet do not crank; they remain in the same relative position.

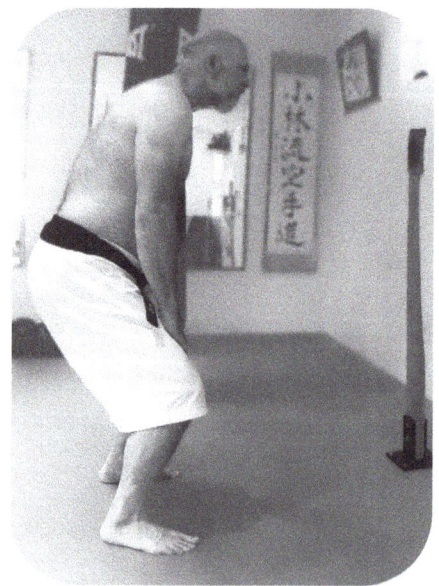

Machiwara Undo always starts and ends by bowing.

マチワラ運動 / Machiwara Undō

Hook punch, Shiko Dachi.

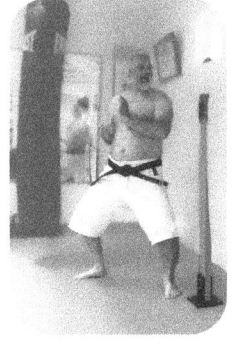 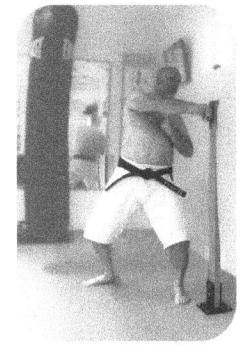

Inside lateral punch, Naihanchi Dachi.

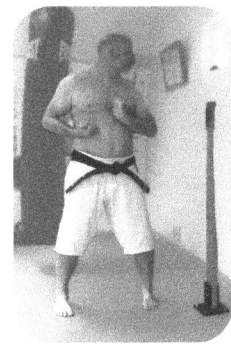 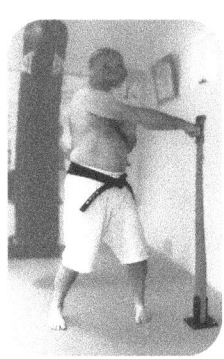 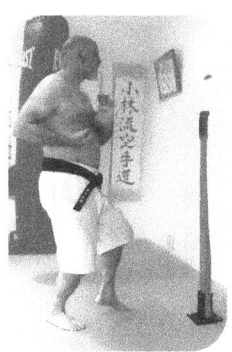

Six methods

Reverse Punch, Neko Ashi Dachi.

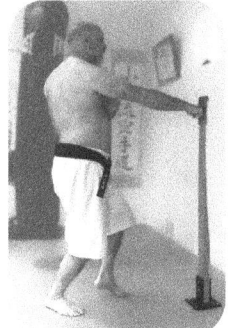 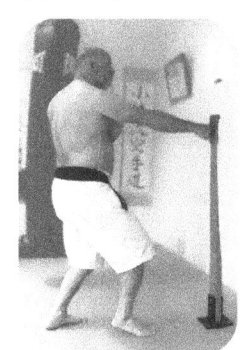

Lunge punch, Neko Ashi Dachi.

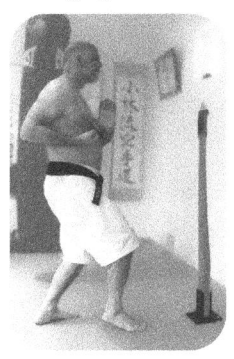 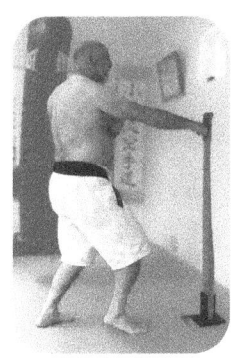

Outside lateral punch, Shizentai.

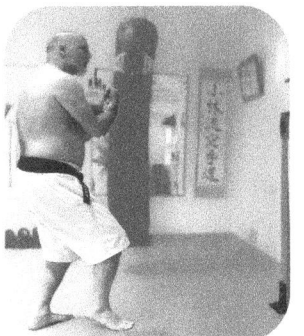 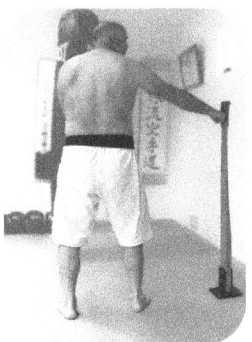

Urate, Naihanchi Dachi.

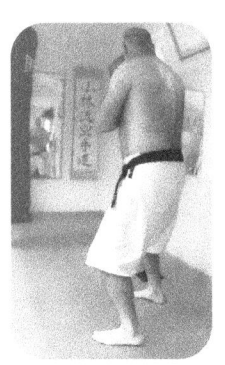 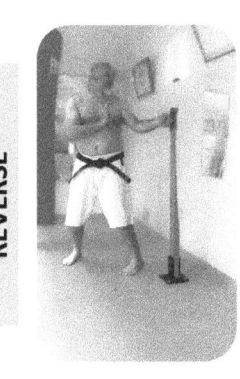

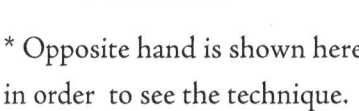

Begin the other side with hook punch.

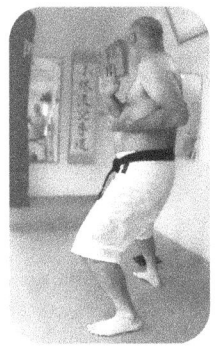 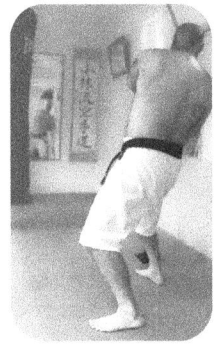

* Opposite hand is shown here in order to see the technique.

マチワラ運動   Machiwara Undō

Machiwara is essential to learning and understanding Onaga No Ti. Onaga sensei shared this text with a select number of students around 2014, in the hope that it would guide them on their path.

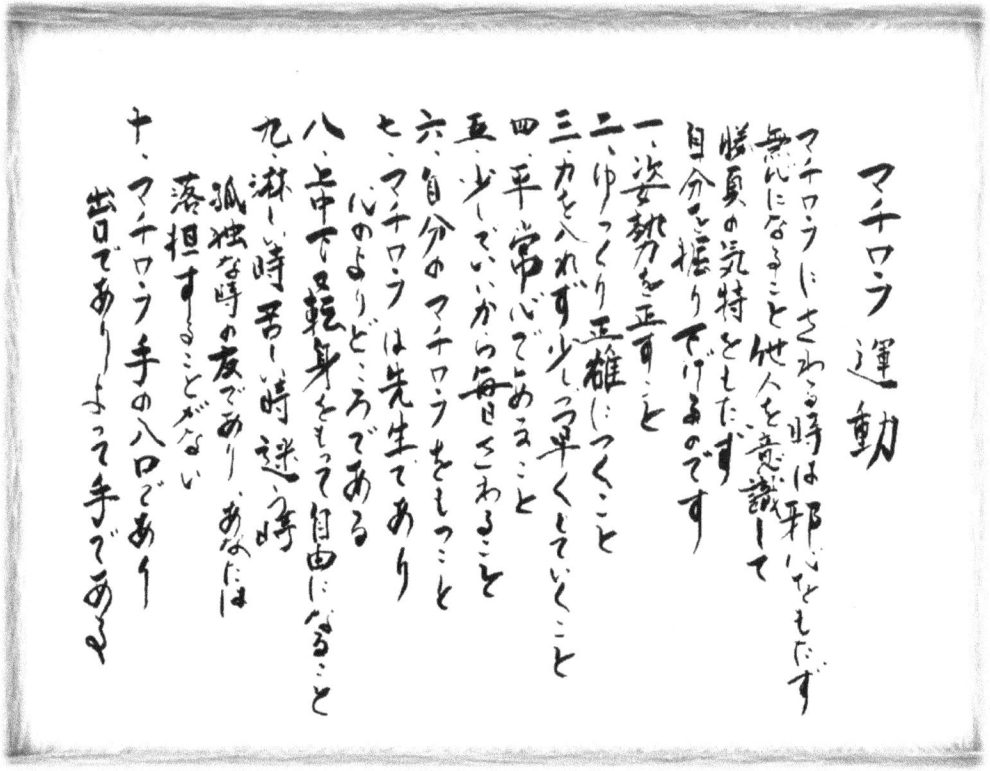

Brushed by: Arakaki Shuniichi   **Translated** by: Masaaki Sato

Machiwara Undo

When touching Machiwara, one should focus on developing the deeper self; no malice, only a still/empty mind. Pay no attention to what others do. Do not approach it in the spirit of competition.

1. Correct the posture and alignment
2. Strike slowly and precisely
3. Increase the speed gradually without the power
4. Remain still of mind
5. Touch Machiwara everyday even a little time
6. Have your own Machiwara
7. Machiwara is a teacher and a pillar of heart
8. Move freely in all directions, upper, middle, and down
9. The Machiwara should be your companion and support you at times of loneliness, loss, or sadness.
10. Machiwara is an entrance and an exit: it is Ti.

<u>Note</u>: Onaga sensei very deliberately uses the word "touch" rather than "strike" when discussing Machiwara practice.

Ashi Waza

A tall Tachi Machiwara (standing Machiwara) is never kicked or pulled towards you. Tachi Machiwara are only ever struck with the hand or elbows. The exception is kicking Machiwara designed to withstand Ashi Waza (leg techniques).

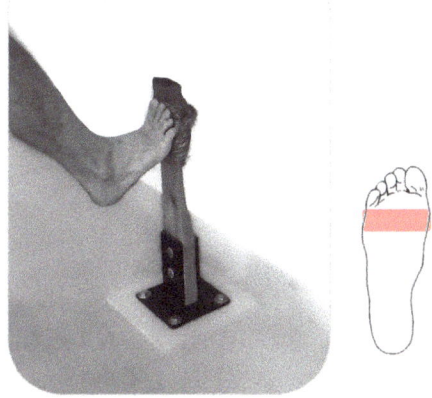

Examples of contact points with the feet on a short kicking Machiwara.

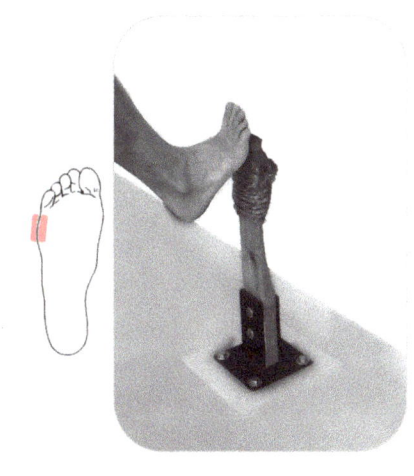
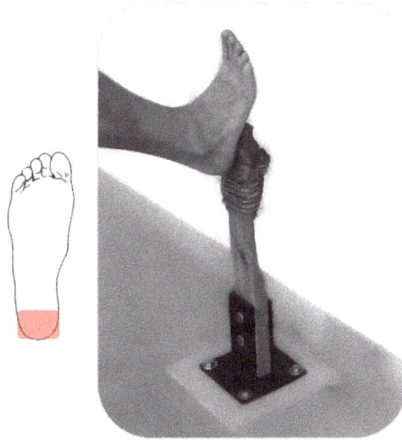
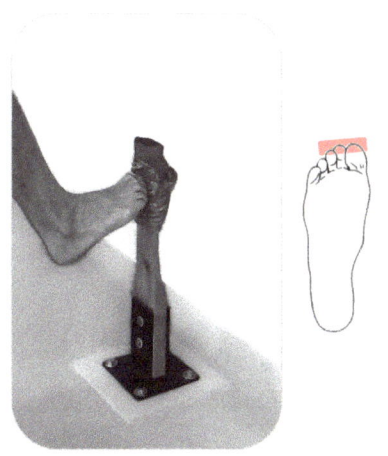
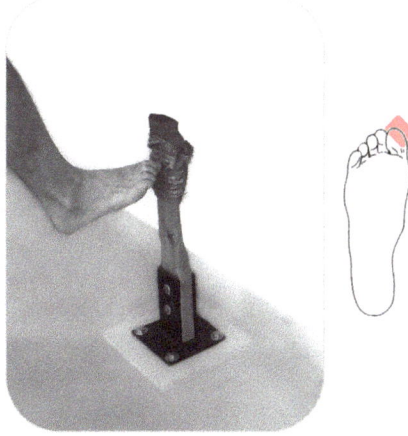

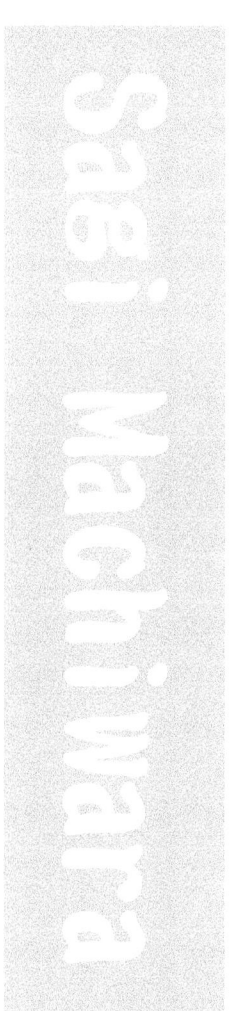

Sagi Machiwara, literally "hanging Machiwara," is perhaps unique to the Onaga Karate Dojo. Similar looking training tools do exist in old Chinese texts, but I've never seen one in any Dojo on Okinawa. That's not to say they don't exist, but I suspect today none do. This Machiwara was originally a log hanging from a tree branch in the outdoor training space in which Onaga sensei first started training as a middle school student.

Even if another Dojo does use these today, the training methods will certainly be completely different, as this is one of the tools that Onaga sensei has dedicated a lot of time and effort into innovating both vertical and horizontal methods, as well as solo and partner exercises.

Sagi Machiwara

サギマチワラ

Sagi Machiwara has 4 basic positions:

1. vertically with the top of the log at eye level
2. horizontal hanging at one's hip level
3. horizontal hanging at one's shoulder level
4. horizontal angled from one's mid-section to the head

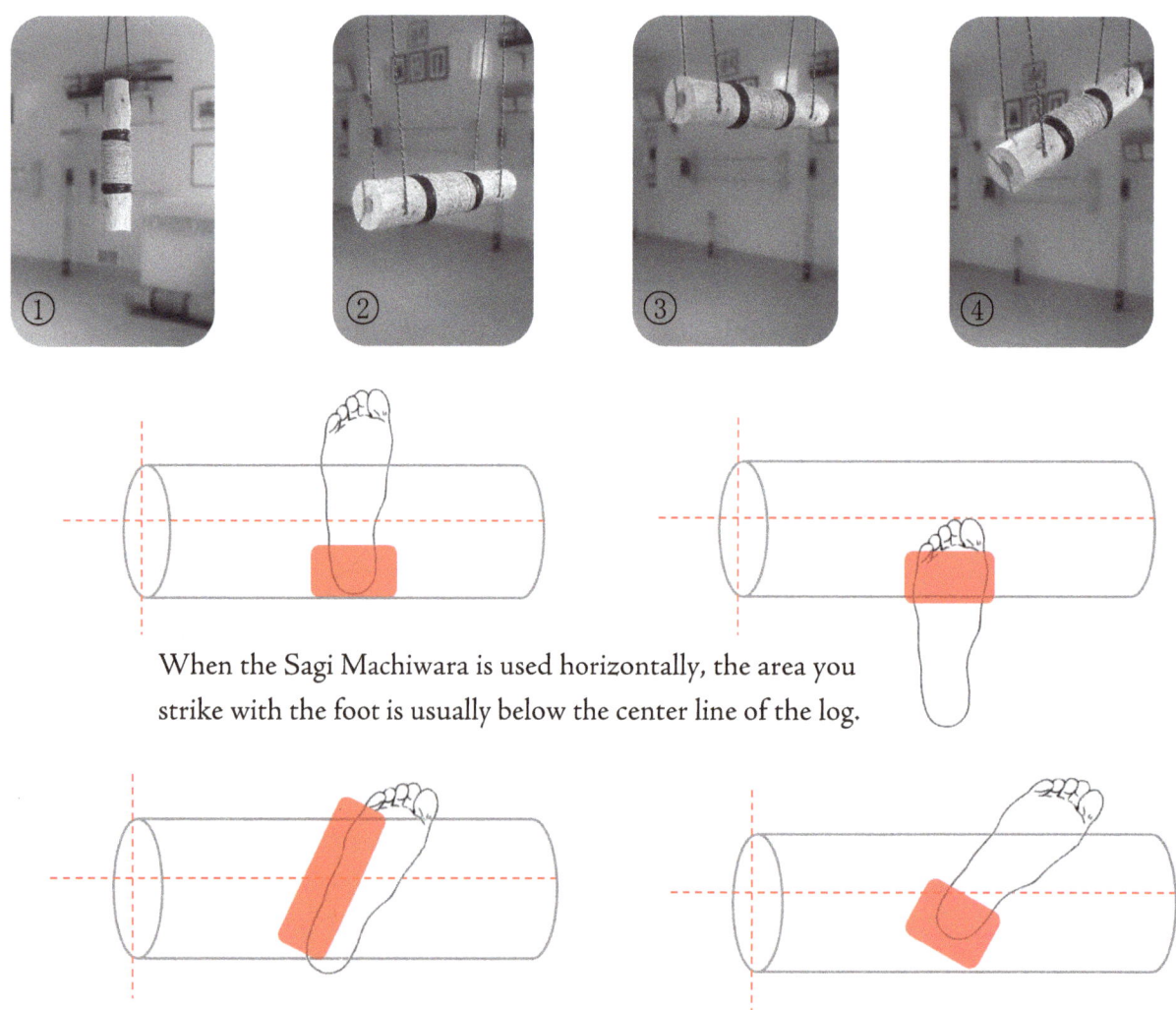

When the Sagi Machiwara is used horizontally, the area you strike with the foot is usually below the center line of the log.

Sagi Machiwara provides a few advantages over other types of training. The swinging movement allows you to train Tenshin as well as striking, with 360° access around the Machiwara. Because it is moving, it requires precision timing and is a reasonable substitute for partner training.

サギマチワラ　　Sagi Machiwara

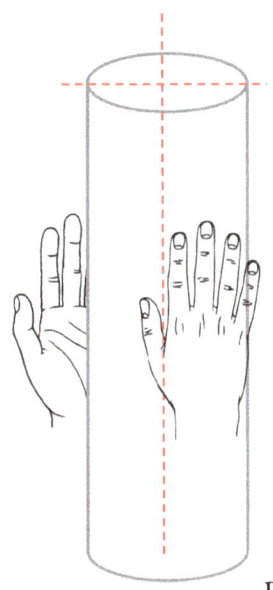
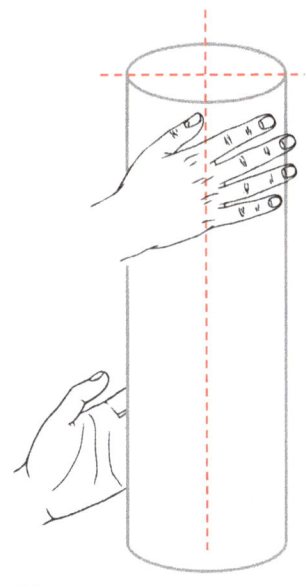

Basic hand positions.

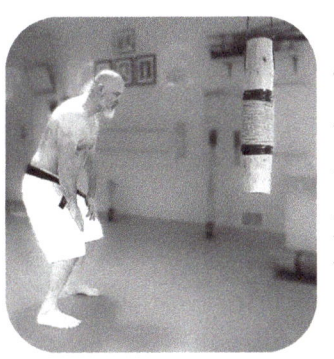

The Machiwara is your partner and your teacher. Like all partner training, begin with a bow.

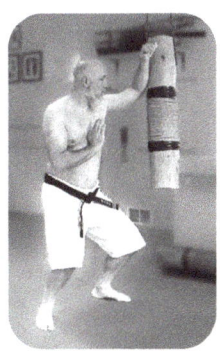
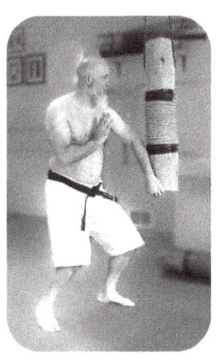
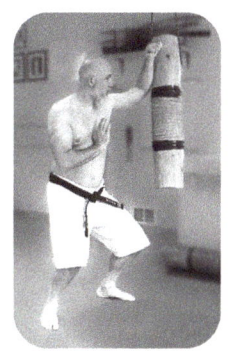

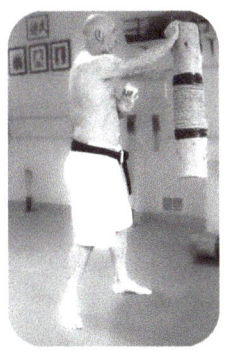
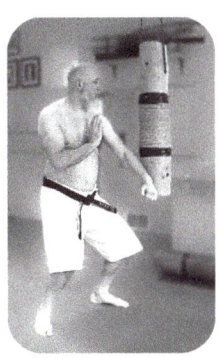
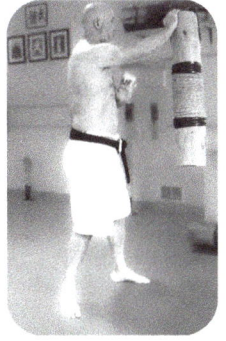
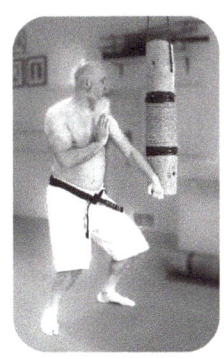

Striking the Machiwara, as well as doing Kukan Tsuki and Kukan Geri while controlling the Machiwara, are the basic forms of practice.

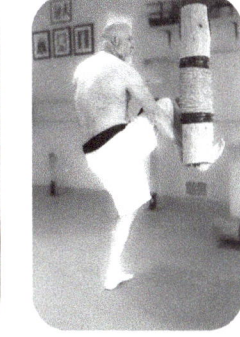
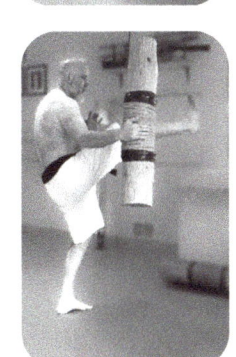
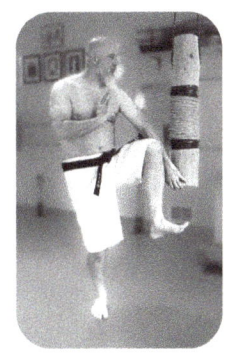
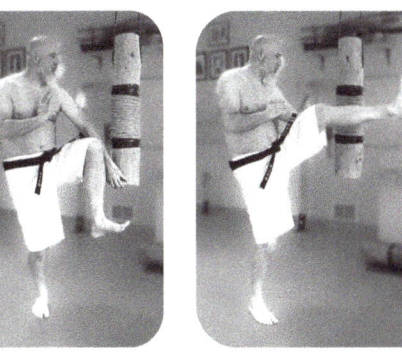

Sagi Machiwara hand positions

サギマチワラ　　Sagi Machiwara

Vertical Sagi Machiwara

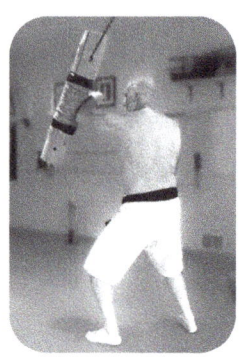 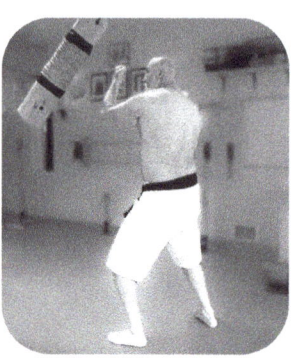 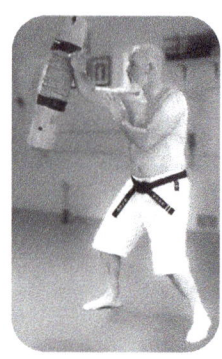

Understanding the Sagi Machiwara: it is not a heavy bag. It is more like a moving wooden dummy. Work on movement, speed, and focus over impact.

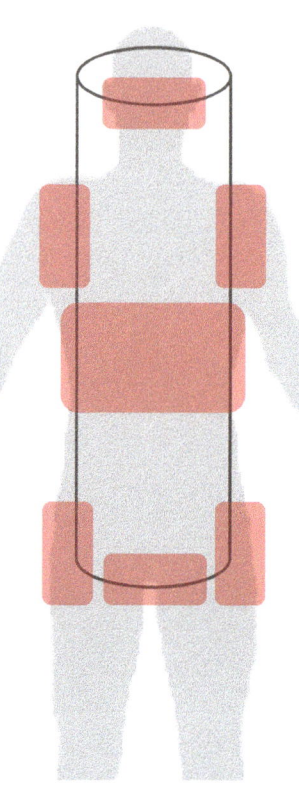

Common targets.

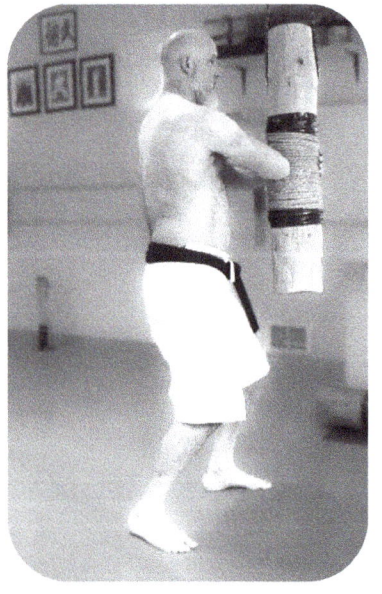

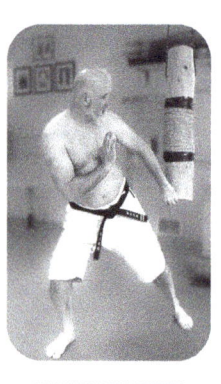 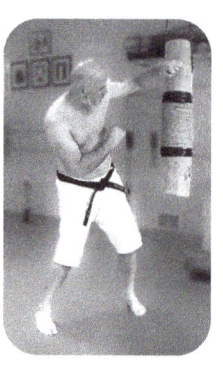 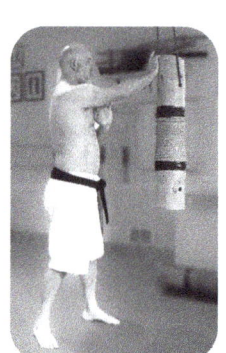
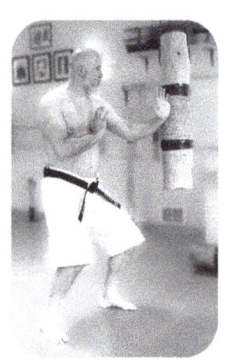 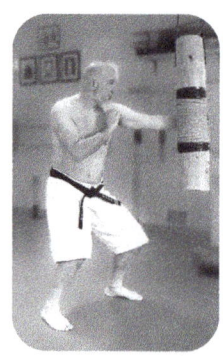 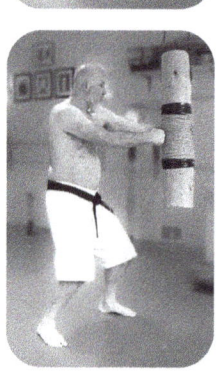

Working from Jigotai, changing the height as well as the direction of the stance.

サギマチワラ / Sagi Machiwara

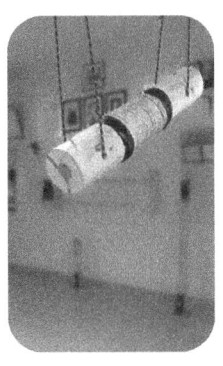
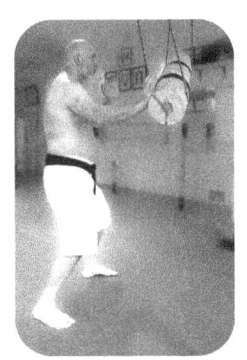
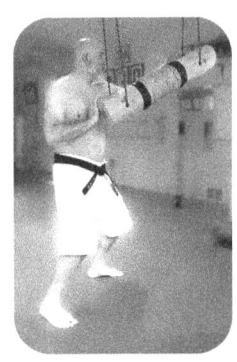
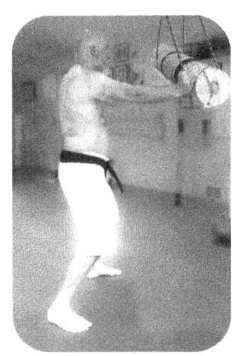

Angled Sagi Machiwara

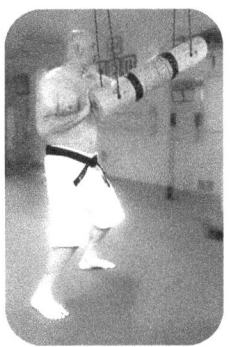
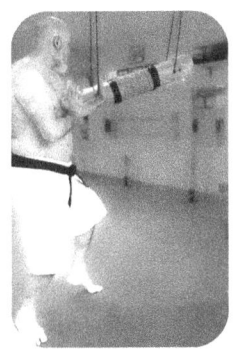
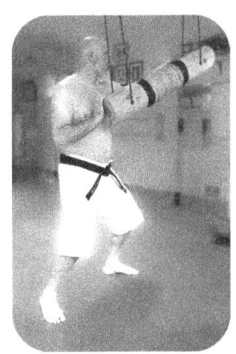

When the Machiwara is horizontal or angled, it represents the opponent's shoulders and arms, or hips and legs.

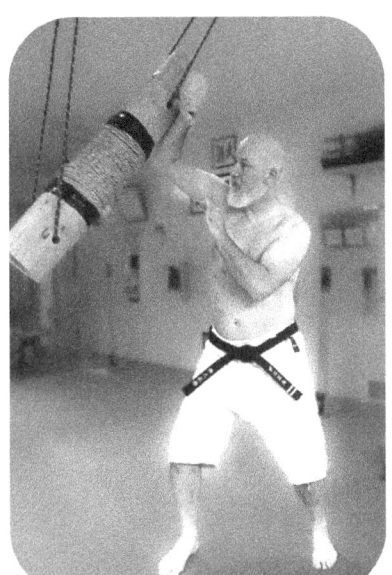
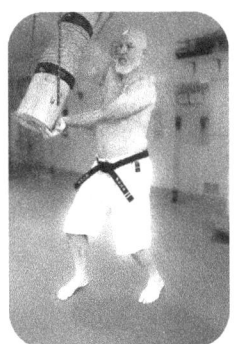
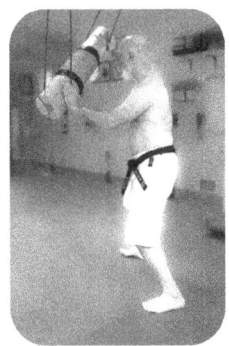
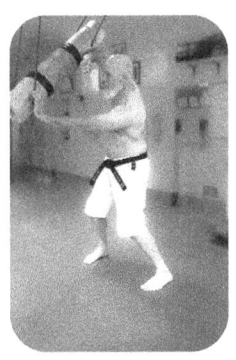
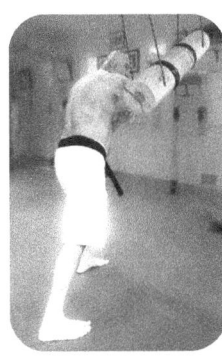
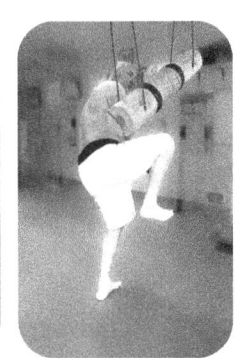
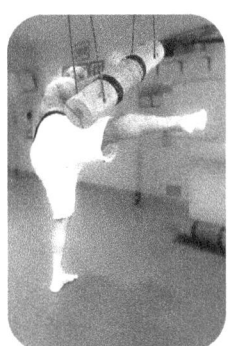

Sagi Machiwara

サギマチワラ

Jodan

Chest or head height.

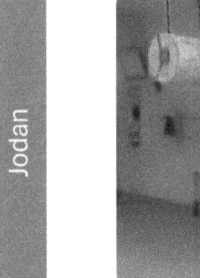
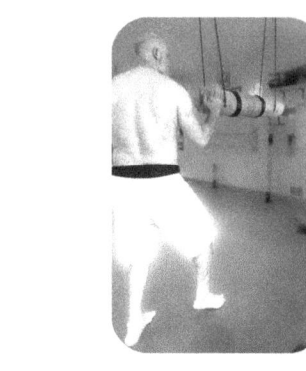
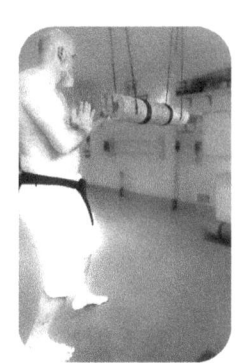

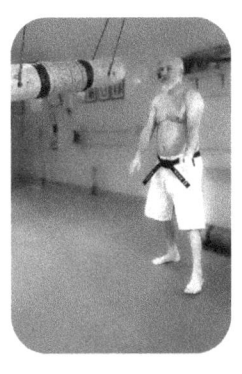
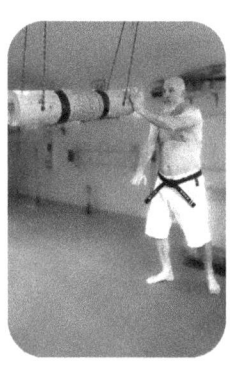
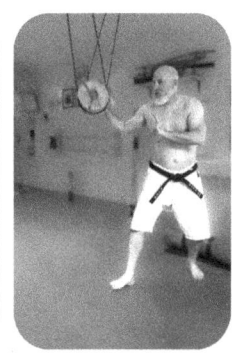
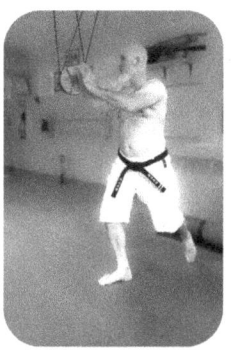
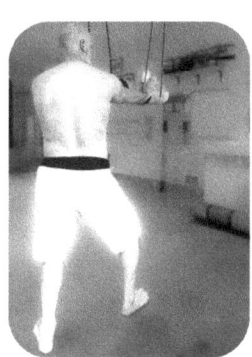

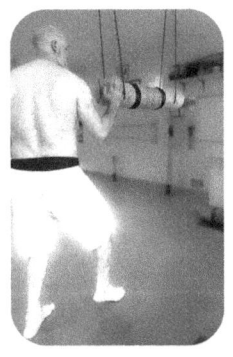
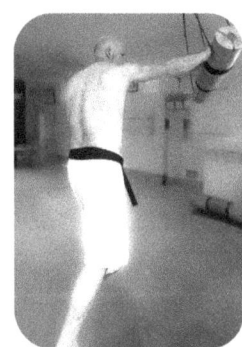
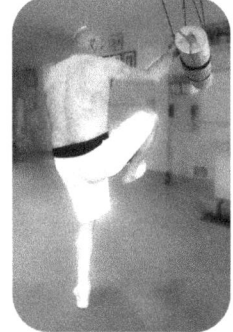
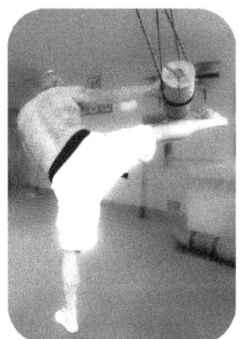

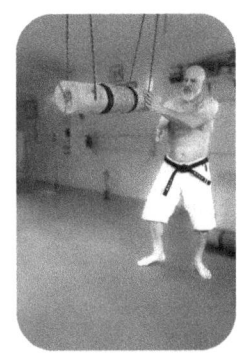
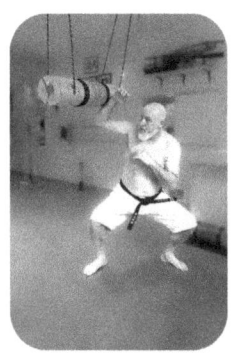
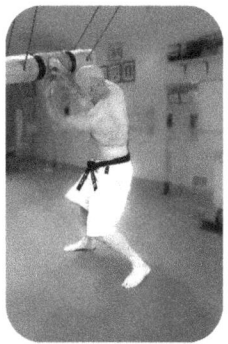
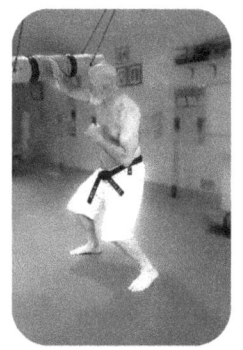

When the Sagi Machiwara is hanging high, it should be thought of as the opponent's shoulders or arm, depending on the exercise.

サギマチワラ　　　　　　　　　　　Sagi Machiwara

Waist height.

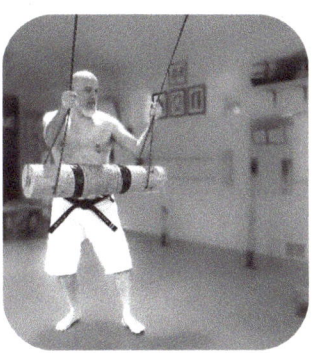 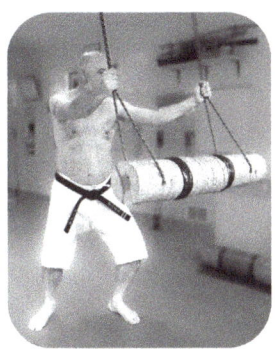

Sagi Machiwara can be practiced as a solitary or partner training method. When done with a partner, the person that would be the "Uke" uses the ropes to move the Machiwara, forward/backward, and twisting to the angles.

Gedan

The are many ways to kick the Sagi Machiwara, but usually the striking surface of the foot is making contact below the centerline of the log.

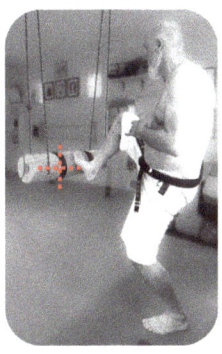 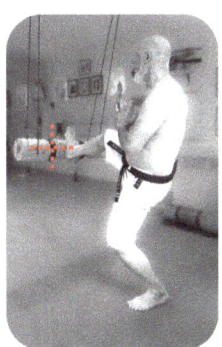 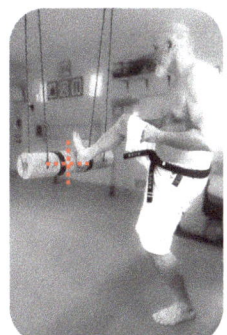 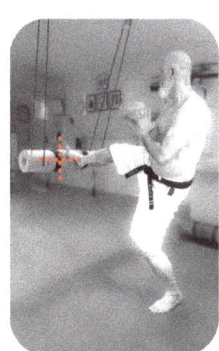 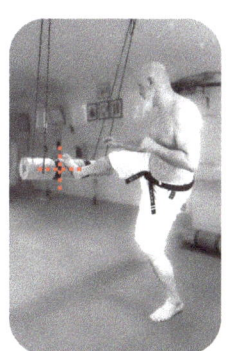

Foot position

Onaga sensei teaching Sagi Machiwara footwork.

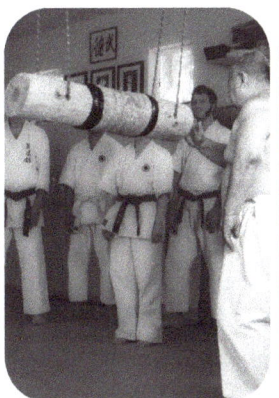 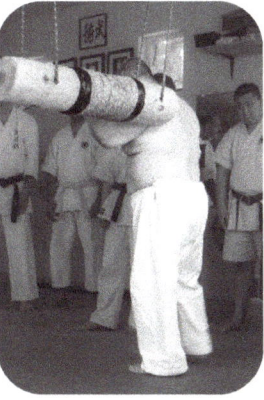 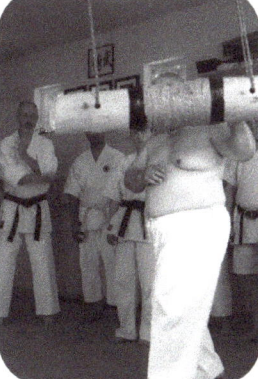 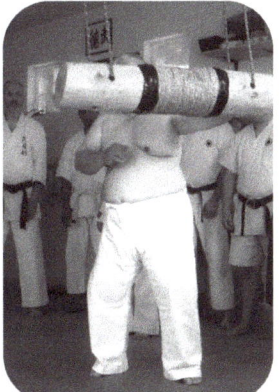 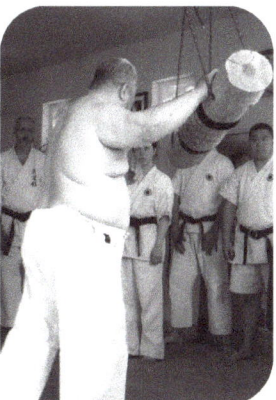

Photos: Guido Penke 2011

Yakusoku Kumite

Yakusoku Kumite (約束組手) is a type of Futari Renshu (二人練習), two-person or partner practice. It is perhaps the most common two-person training for junior students because the defender knows what to expect, the attacker is able to strike hard and fast, allowing the defender to experience more realistic speed and power. The counter attacks: Tsuki, Keri, Empi, and Urate are further combined with In and Yo, and the 7 Tenshin patterns.

Yakusoku Kumite

Each of the Yakusoku Kumite in our Dojo begin in the same way, with the Uke striking, and the Tori using Tenshin and then covering across the body and controlling the attack.

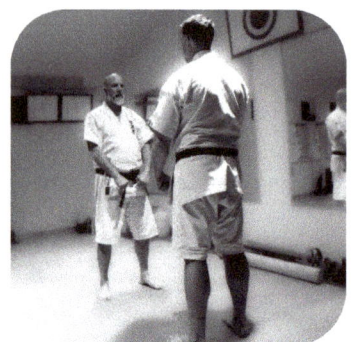
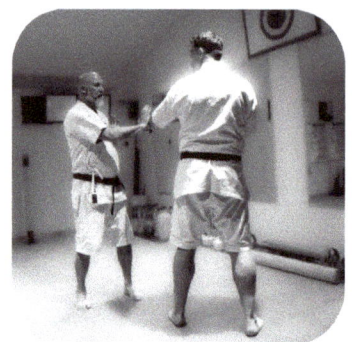
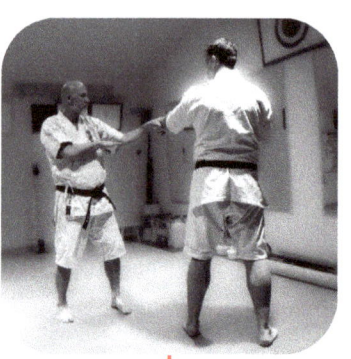

After the attack is controlled, one of the 4 counters is applied from the outside, Yo position.

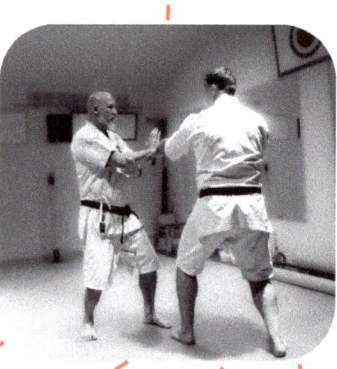

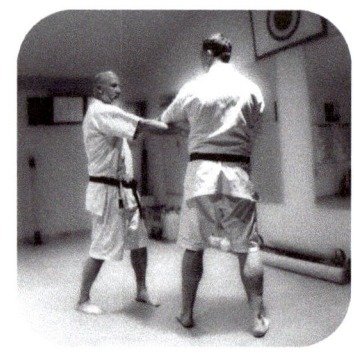
1. Tsuki

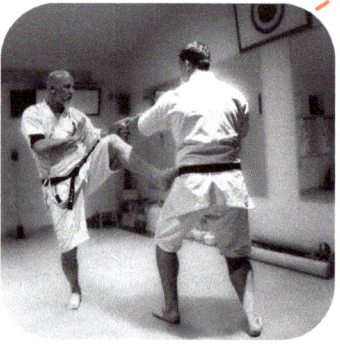
2. Keri

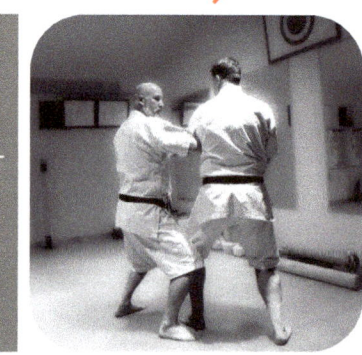
3. Empi

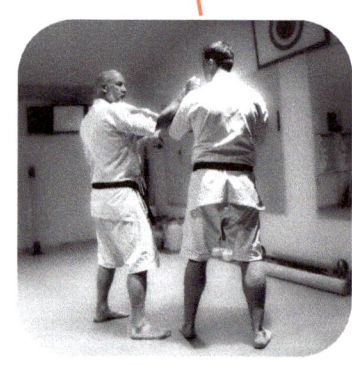
4. Urate

Yakusoku Kumite

The same pattern is used when the Uke attacks from the other side, although the attacker switches sides the Tori does not, resulting in the Tori getting the inside path.

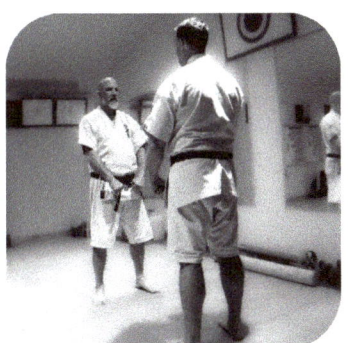 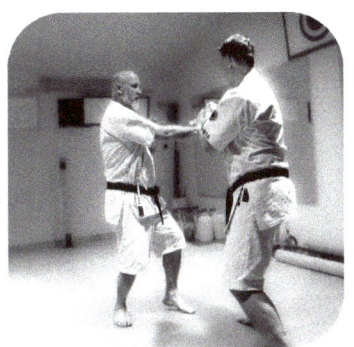 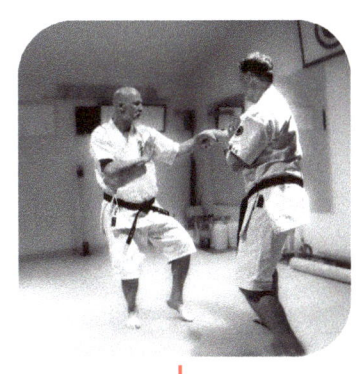

Unlike the Yo techniques, when doing In some counter attacks result in less desirable positioning and are modified to be more practical.

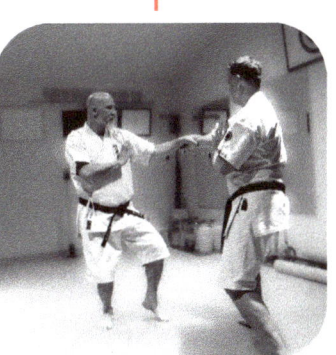

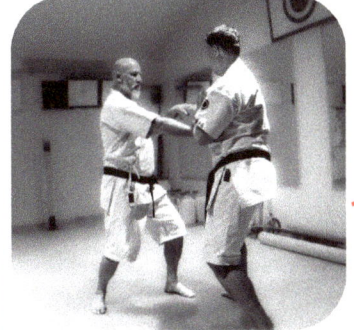
1. Tsuki

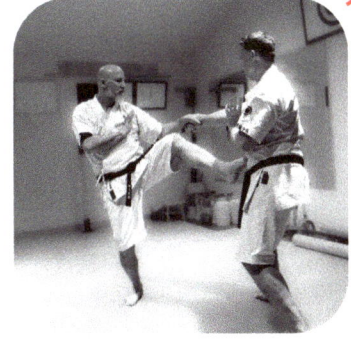
2. Keri

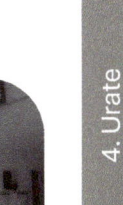
3. Empi

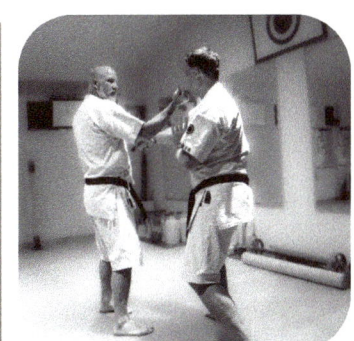
4. Urate

Empi is changed to Kake Age Jichi (rising hook strike).

Yakusoku Kumite

Here the same pattern is repeated with the Uke thrusting out with a Shomen Mae Geri. The Tori does Tenshin to the side, covers across to hook the leg.

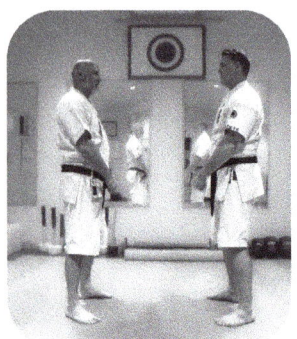 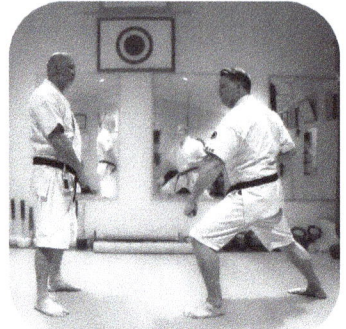 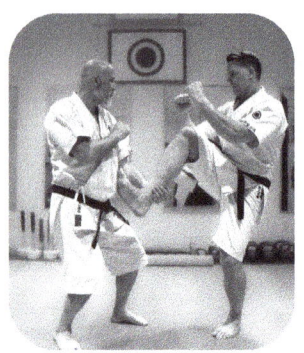

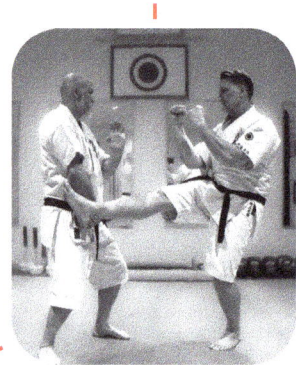

In the same way that the Uke could attack either In or Yo with the arms, both are valid options for the kicks.

After the attack is controlled, one of the 4 counters is applied from the outside. The targets for the counter attacks have changed slightly as a result of the attacker's posture after kicking.

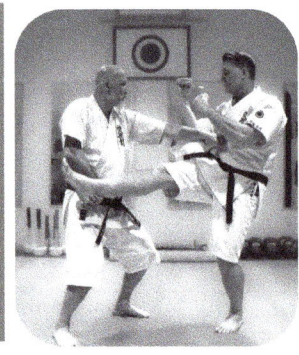

1. Tsuki

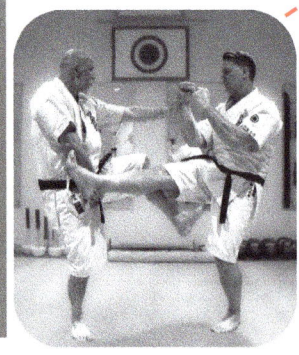

2. Keri

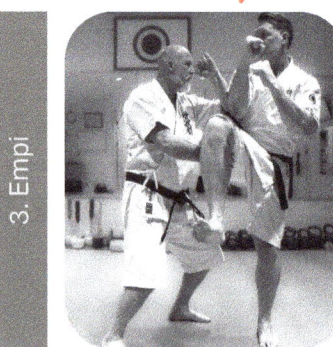

3. Empi

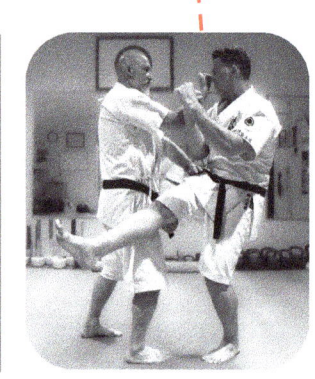

4. Urate

二人練習　　Futari Renshu

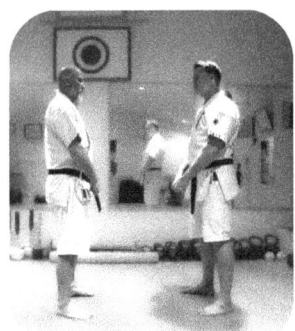 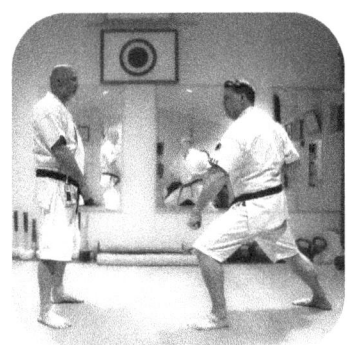 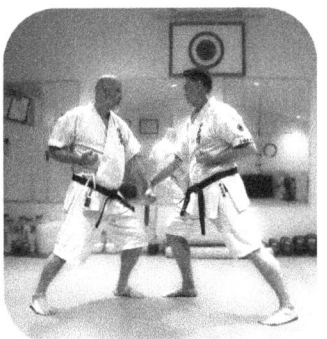 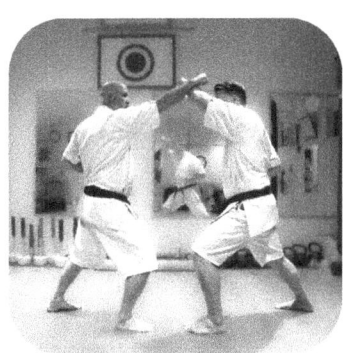

There are countless variations of prearranged partner practice. The most basic patterns of Futari Renshu (partner practice) are done in Zenkutsu Dachi, and Mashomen (straight forward). The number of steps taken by either the Uke or Tori are agreed upon prior to training.

Uke: 受け Literally the receiver, which is confusing when translated, but it implies they will receive the technique being practiced by their partner. The Uke is a training partner/tool.

Tori: 取り is the person who "takes" the attack and successfully completes the counter. The Uke is present to allow the Tori to have an opponent with whom to practice the technique.

In the Dojo we often use the term "Uke" but seldom say "Tori." The more structured and standardized 2 person patterns are the Yakusoku Kumite. These can be done in Shizentai (natural stance) moving into Neko Ashi Dachi or can start directly from Jigotai, depending on the student's level.

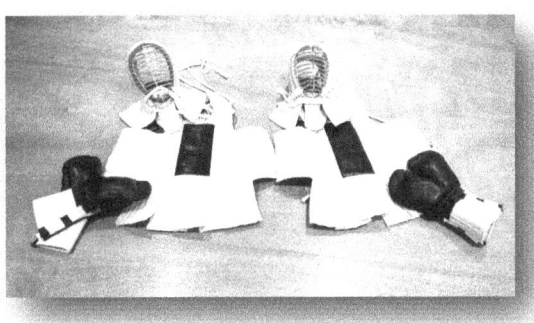

Bogu—body armor made from modified kendo helmets. Cotton, leather and bamboo chest plates, padded leather gloves.

Free sparring with Bogu, another form of partner practice, is primarily used to learn what it feels like to be on the receiving end of a strike. This is not to develop "resistance" to being hit, but to understand the power necessary to attain "Atifa."

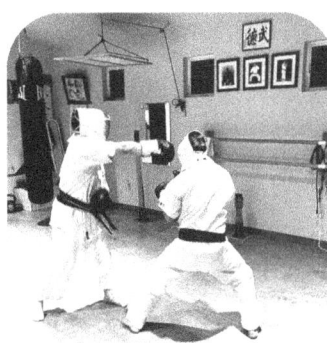 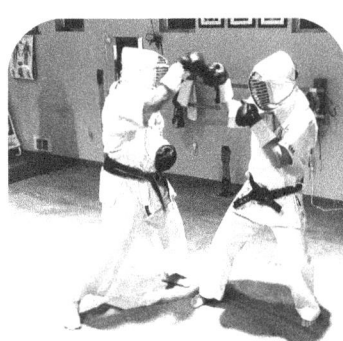 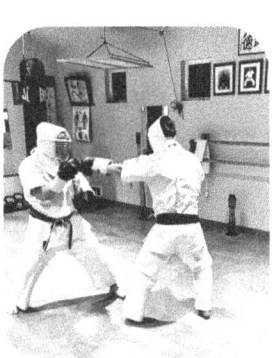

Bogu Jiyu Kumite

二人練習　　　　　　　　　　Futari Renshu

Other examples of partner practice are Kakie and Irikumi.

Kakie

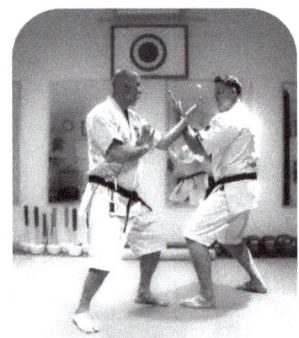 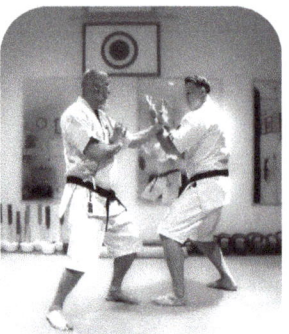 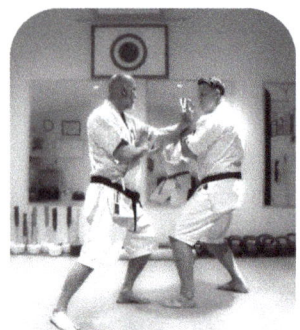 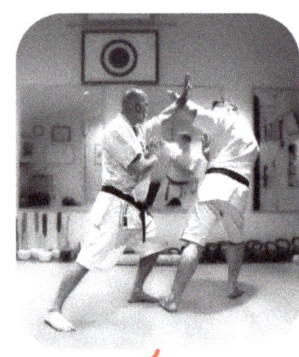

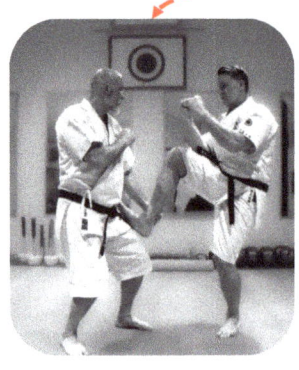 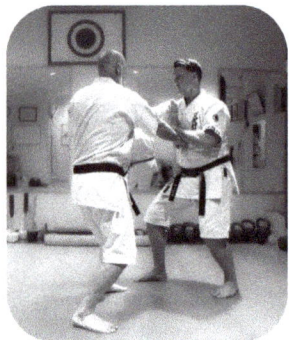 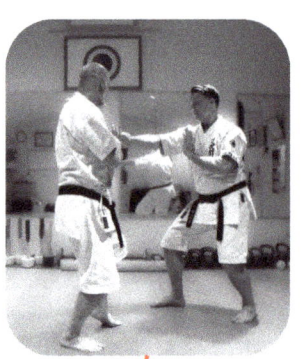

Kakie, when done at speed and without following any pattern, is the most advanced and risky training method.

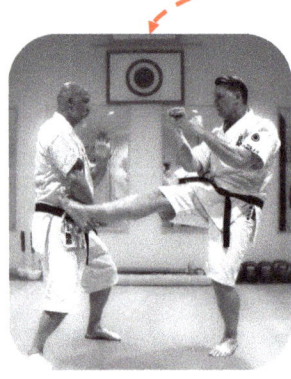 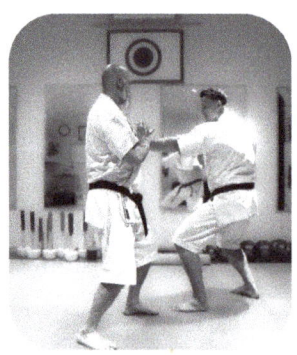 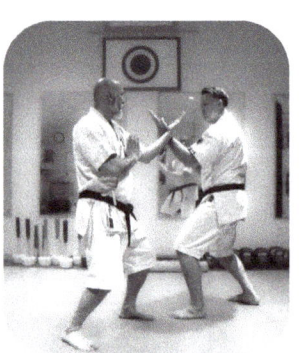

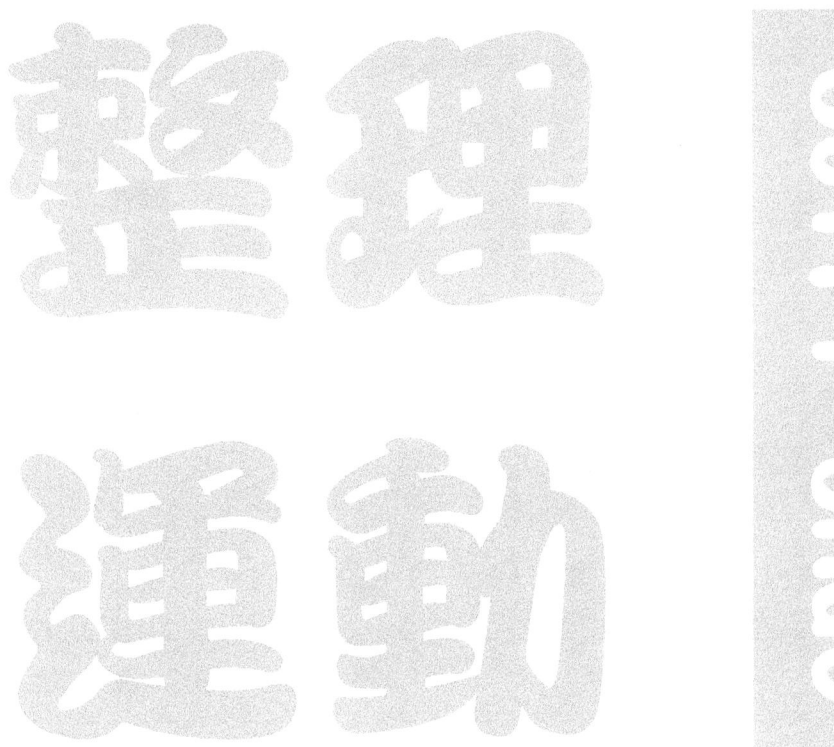

Seiri Undo (整理運動) is most commonly translated as a simple "cooldown exercise," although Seiri has a much deeper meaning in Zen training. It is done at the end of class, often with the lights off. The term is made of two ideas: "Seiri" which means to organize or arrange and "Undo" meaning exercise. Although used primarily as a means to get the heart rate down and relax the muscles, the other important aspect of Seiri Undo is to compose oneself before concluding the training session. Students should put their Keikogi (稽古着, practice uniform) tops back on if they had been removed during training, or take the opportunity to arrange themselves by straightening the Obi (帯, belt) and Keikogi prior to bowing Shomen, to the instructor, and to their peers.

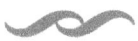

整理運動　　　　　　　　　　　　　　Seiri Undō

After the initial sets of "hops" which are done in silence, all students are expected to count out each movement in counts of 8 in Japanese.

Hops

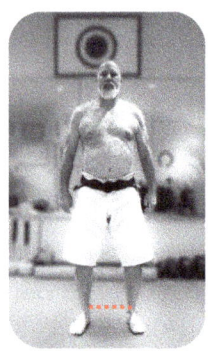
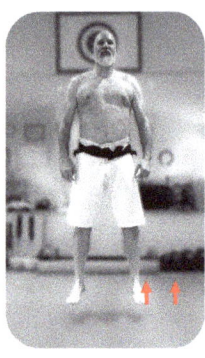
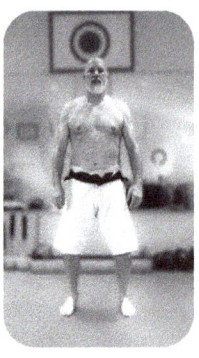
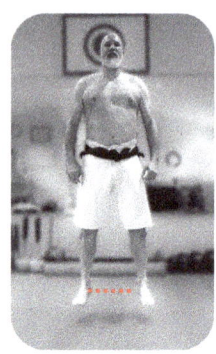

Toes up, feet flat while hopping.

Land quietly.

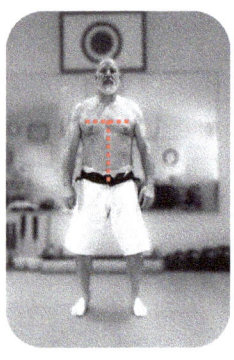
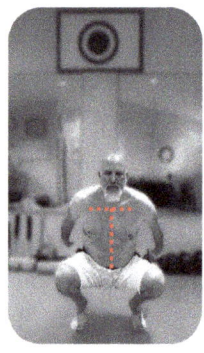
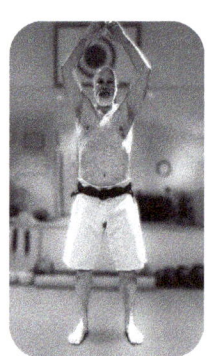
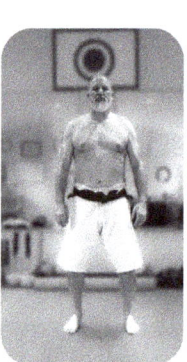

Chest

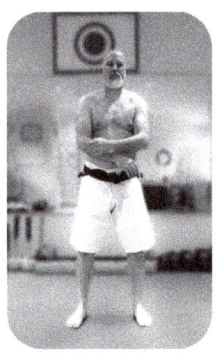
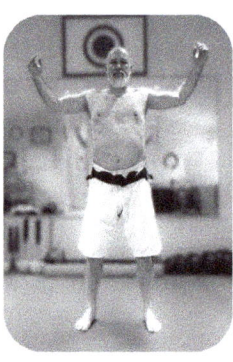
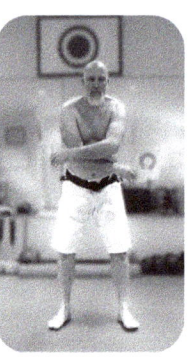
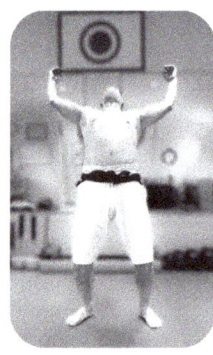
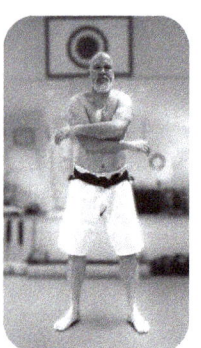

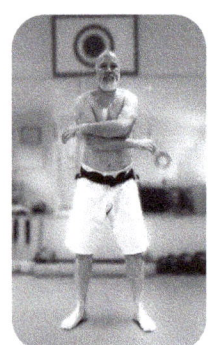
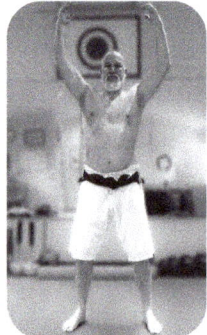
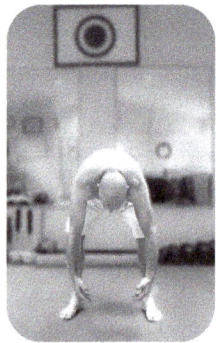
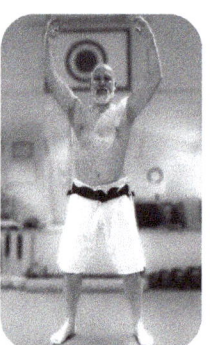
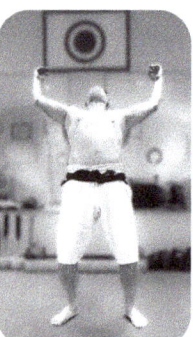

整理運動　　　　Seiri Undō

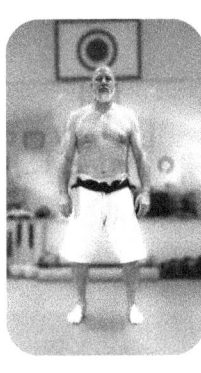 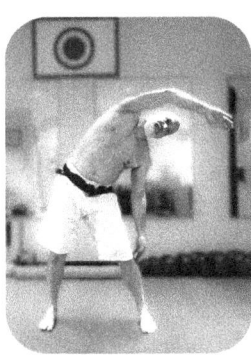 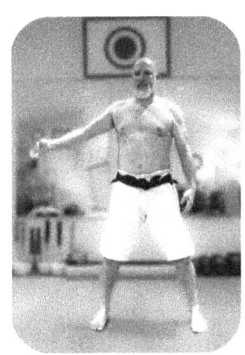

Many of the exercises in the Seiri Undo are repeated from the Yobi Undo and are done the same way as at the start of class.

Lateral tilt

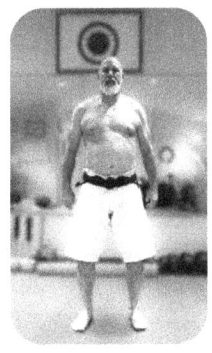 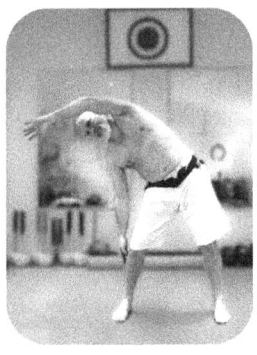 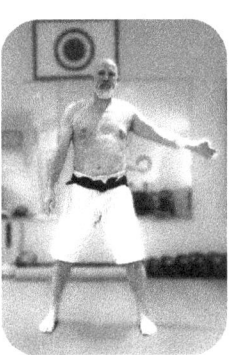

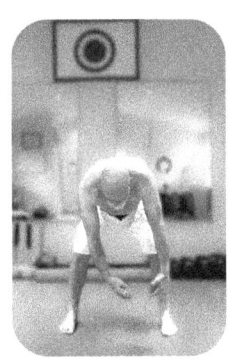 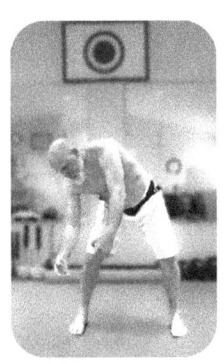 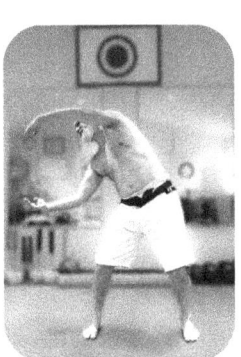 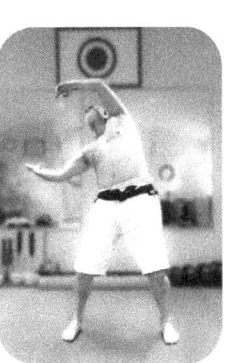 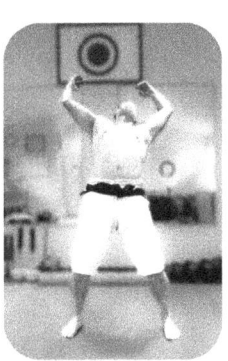

Torso rotations

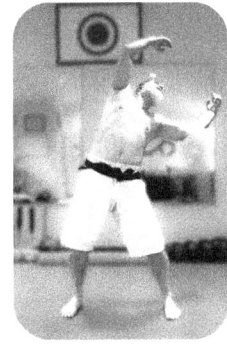 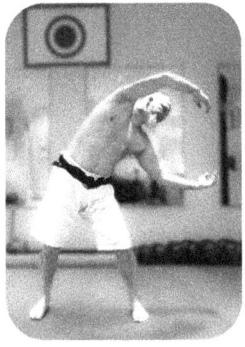 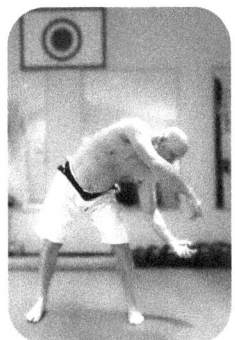 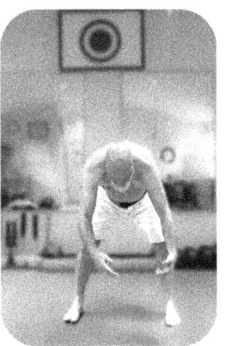

The eyes follow the rotation of the torso.

整理運動　　　　　　　　　　　　Seiri Undō

Torso recline

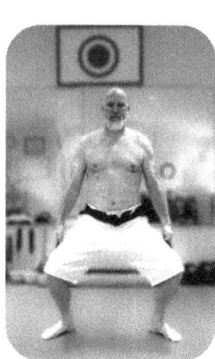 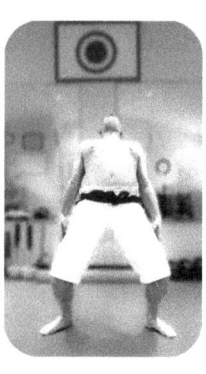 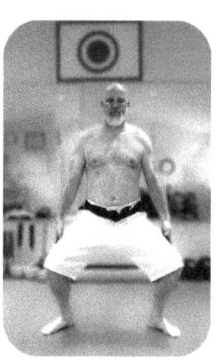

Push the hips forward to cause the shoulders, neck, and head to lean back.

Torso twists

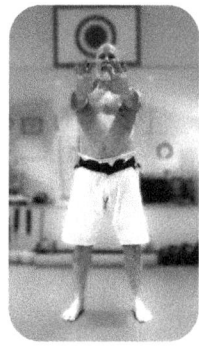 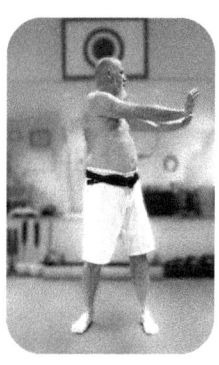 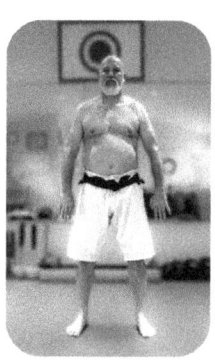 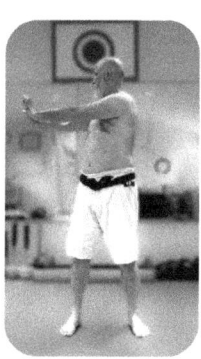 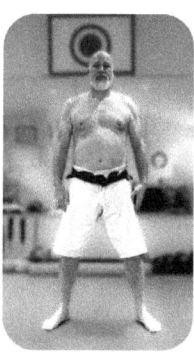

Breathing

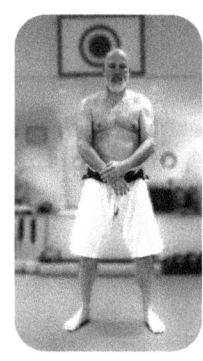 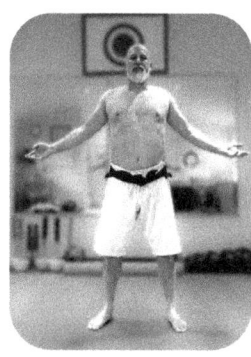 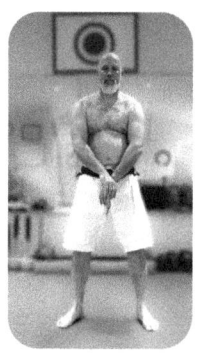 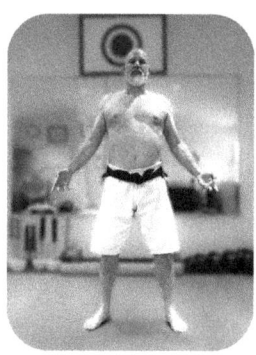

Expand to inhale; collapse the chest to exhale.

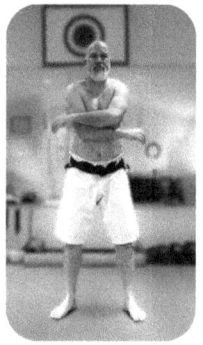 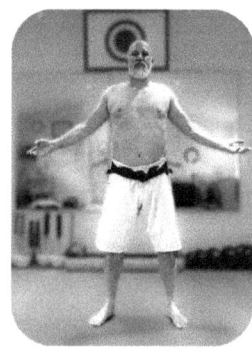 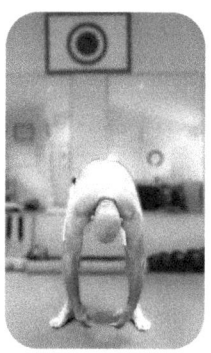 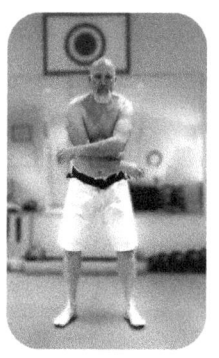

Finish exhaling slowly at the bottom, then wait with the breath paused before expanding up.

Seiri Undō

整理運動

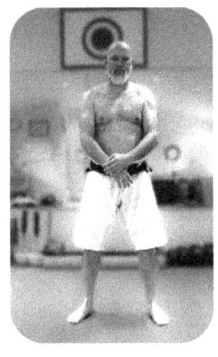 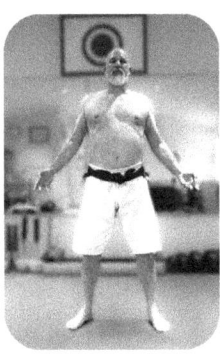 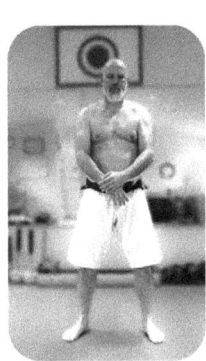 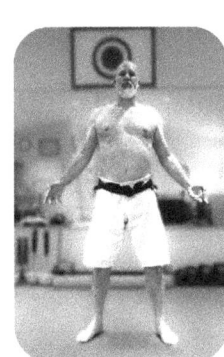

Quick, shallow breaths.

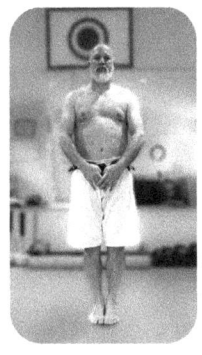 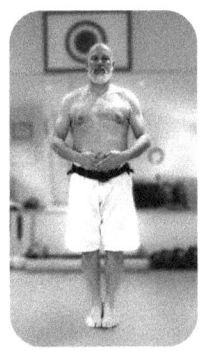 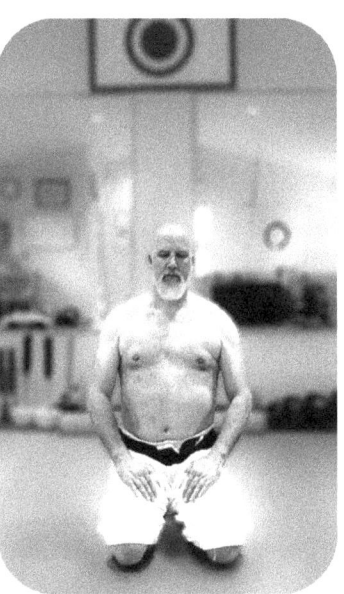

Mokuso (meditation) standing, then in Seiza.

Mokuso

Seiri Undo is usually done with the lights off, if training indoors. Once the teacher instructs "Mokuso Yame," meditation is finished, then students will form lines to bow out of class.

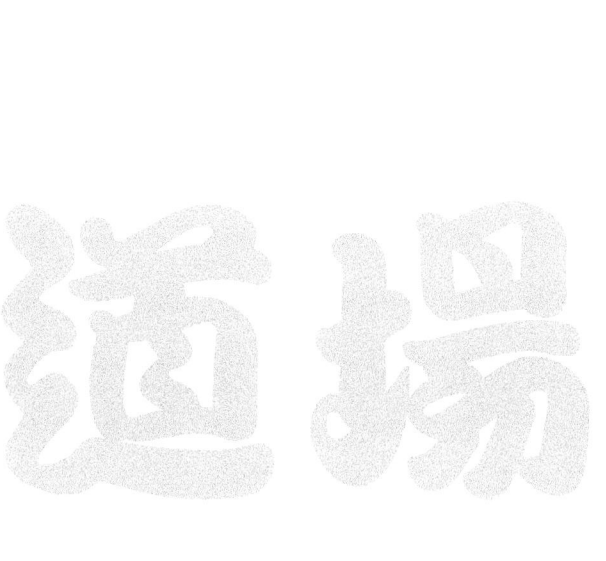
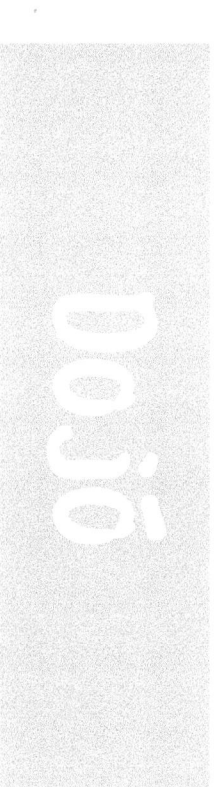

A Dojo is not a studio, or a gym, or a training hall. A Dojo (道場) is where you learn and practice "the way," Do (道). It can be indoors or outdoors, dirt floor, or hardwood. Where you bow, pay respect, and apply yourself to learning —that is the Dojo. The character for Jo (場) is commonly used in the context of a scene in a play or movie, or even when referring to an academic field or area. It is best to think of it less as a place and more as a situation. It is the setting where you learn, train, teach, or practice the way.

There is no need for a Dojo to be a physical building, although most are today. Students would often train in the teacher's yard, or sometimes at a grave site. What makes a place a Dojo is the attitude you bring and the teaching and learning that takes place. As a result, the act of bowing is what turns a room from a classroom or gym into a Dojo, or a patch of dirt into a Dojo. But when it is a permanent physical space dedicated to Karate, there are a few norms for what makes a "traditional" Dojo in the modern era.

Once in the Dojo, whether indoors or outdoors, when practicing Hojo Undo, Kigu Undo or essentially any practice, never focus on completing a certain number of repetitions. Instead, focus on how much time is spent on an exercise or technique, not on the number of repetitions completed. The intention is not to reach a specific number, but to always execute the next movement to the best of one's ability. Always "one more," regardless of how long it's been.

Although practice can take place any time of day, there are generally two types of practice: Asa Geiko (朝稽古, or morning practice), and Ban Geiko (晩稽古, evening practice). Of course, the obvious difference is as the names imply, but the important difference is the type of exercises practiced. In the morning, training is usually lighter, more technical, and more about internalizing the concepts and muscle memory, while evening practice is physical, heavy training, both in effort and spirit, usually done at a pace that would be difficult to last more than a few hours.

During evening class, students are often expected to go until exhaustion, to reach a point where simply powering through using muscle strength just isn't feasible, and one begins to understand how to leverage the technique and body mechanics to compensate for the lack of strength brought on by fatigue. Once a student is able to understand how to use the hips, Gammaku, or Tenshin to execute the technique, in spite of the lack of physical strength, one is expected to retain that and then apply the same body mechanics when back at full strength.

As mentioned previously, it's best not to focus on the number of repetitions. There are famous teachers who pride themselves on executing two thousand, or even ten thousand, strikes in a row. The problem is that when the goal is reaching a number, everything else is sacrificed. Technique, breathing, and power all become less important than reaching the number. When doing consecutive Rensoku Tsuki (連続) practice, what we usually refer to as Kukan Tsuki, air striking, (空間突き) or air kicking, Kukan Geri, (空間蹴り) always focus on "one more" strike, as hard, as fast, and with the best possible technique. The last technique in the series should be as high quality as the first, if not better, so students shouldn't worry about how many are completed, but rather how long they can do their best for. Students should always find a way to do one more.

During class, students shouldn't speak, certainly shouldn't socialize, and should only speak when addressed. Of course, if a student has been asked to help or teach someone, then speaking is required. The same is true if one has a question, but small talk or sidebar conversations are just not appropriate during class or while others are practicing in the Dojo.

Never stand and watch unless instructed to; while in the Dojo, you need to be applying effort. If you are watching to learn something being taught that is one thing; stand upright, don't lean on anything, and keep your arms at your sides, not on your hips or crossed at your chest. You should never be a spectator, just watching to take a rest, while others practice. If you need to step aside during class, or if you are unable to take part in class for some reason, then obtain permission to sit on the sidelines. Students do not get to step in and out of class at their leisure.

There is an important distinction made between a student and a disciple (Seito versus Deshi). Often these words get loosely translated as "student", but just like in English, there is a nuanced difference. Deshi, strictly speaking, should be disciple and is often considered as close as family. The bond is strengthened when the Deshi understands the concept of Giri (孝), filial piety, duty, burden of obligation, and in return the teacher has committed to ensuring that the Deshi finds their way on the path ahead of them. Seito is what most westerners understand when they hear the word "student."

Dōjo

道場

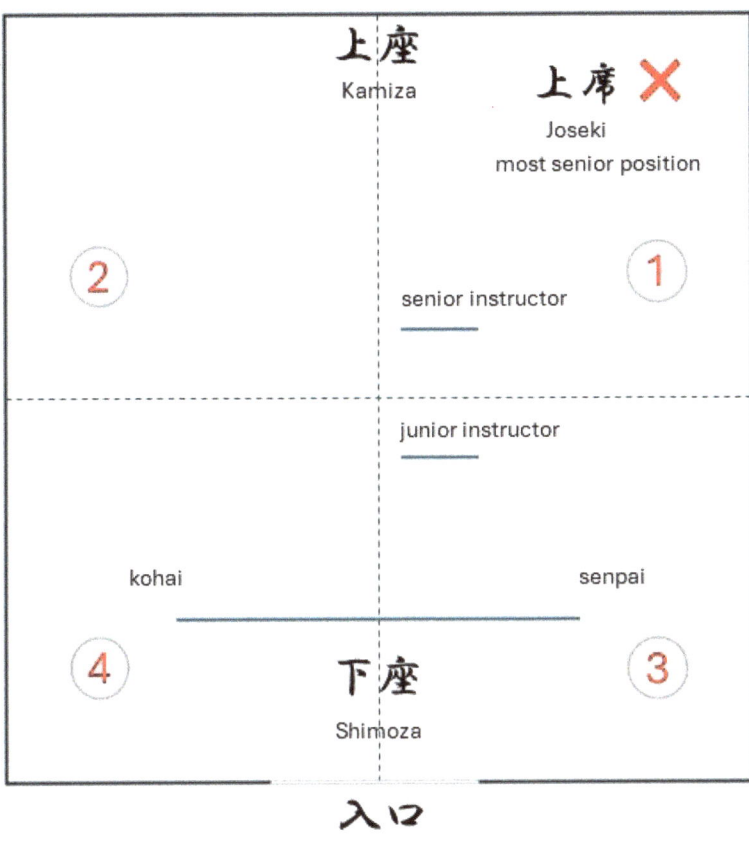

The Dojo is divided into quadrants. The most senior position in the Dojo at the front righthand side, quadrant 1, and the lowest ranked area of the Dojo in quadrant 4.

Depending on the seniority of the instructor, they may choose to stand either on the front or back half of the Dojo when bowing for the start or end of class.

Students will claim a spot to the rear left and wait to be "pushed" up as Kohai fill in the most junior training space.

The Dojo entrance is typically placed at the rear so that you face the Kamiza as you enter.

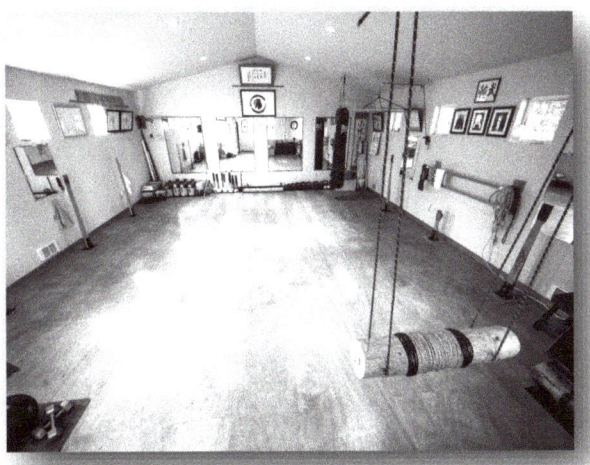

View as you enter the Dojo with the Shomen directly ahead. You can see the Dojo Kun at the very top, center.

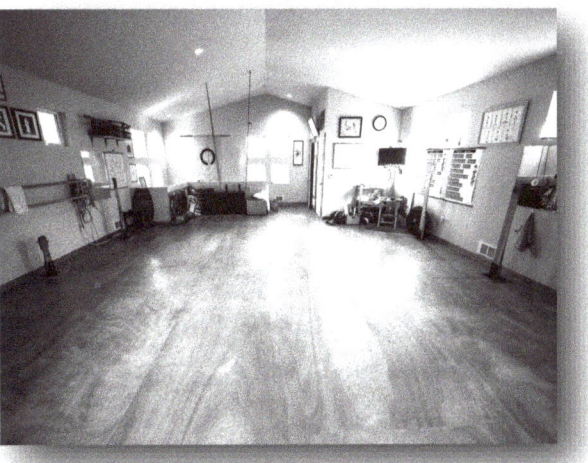

The view from the front of the Dojo towards the Shimoza, rear of the Dojo.

Name, crests, logos

"Everyone" has some idea or understanding of what we mean when we say Karate (空手). They may or may not know the literal translation to be "empty hand" or know that it came about as a political accommodation made during the ultra-nationalistic period of early 20th century, when the Japanese nationalists, in an attempt to erase, or at least obscure, the connection between Okinawa and China, replaced the term Tode (唐手), meaning Chinese hand, which was also read as "Karate," with empty hand.

What is less clear to most people entering a Karate Dojo for the first time are the various styles, or schools. Most people simple say "Karate." Our Dojo is the Shinjinbukan Shorin-ryu Matsu Mizumi (Pine Lake) Shibu. Karate is the art, Shinjinbukan is the school, Shorin-ryu is the style, and Matsu Mizumi (Pine Lake) is the name of the Shibu, or branch, within the association.

Shorin-ryu, small forest lineage, is one of three major 20th century Karate styles on Okinawa. Named and founded by Chibana Choshin (1885-1969), who referred to his Dojo as the "Daiichi Dojo." His senior student, Higa Yuchoku (1910-1994), went on to establish the Kyudokan school of Shorin-ryu, which continues to exist today in Naha, Okinawa, and around the world. This is where Onaga Yoshimitsu sensei trained for over 30 years and lived as an Uchideshi (内弟子, closed door disciple) for over 13 years. While at the Kyudokan, he taught classes at the Hombu (本部, headquarters), as well as at a branch Dojo at a local high school. In 1988/89, Onaga sensei opened his own Dojo, separate from

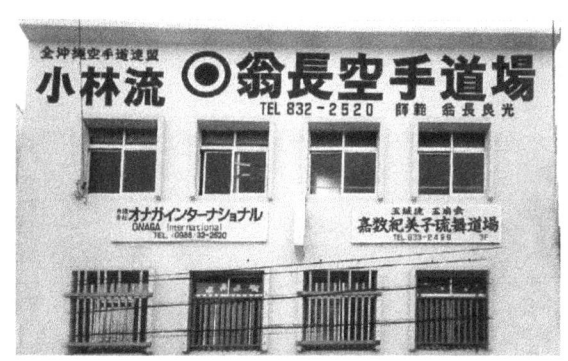

the Kyudokan, and for the first 12 years or so after opening his own Dojo, until the turn of the millennium, the Dojo was simply referred to as the Onaga Karate Dojo (翁長空手道場), as seen in the photograph. The style is Shorin-ryu (小林流) and the Kanji next to the crest reads "Onaga Karate Dojo." The name changed for the celebration of the new millennium when Onaga sensei formally adopted the name **Shinjinbukan,** which had been his intention all along, as evidenced by the fact that the Dojo Kun which hung at the front of the Dojo "spelled out" Shin- Jin- Bu- Kan.

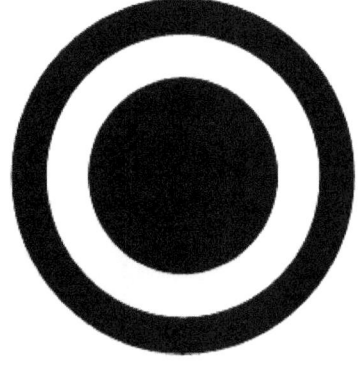

The Onaga Karate Dojo adopted the two tone crest from the very start. Designed by Onaga sensei, it's worn on the Keikogi and was also hung as a flag in the Dojo. The crest shape symbolizes the softness, smoothness of the human heart. The lack of sharp, jagged points or angles is what we should be striving for during training.

Although often mistaken as 3 different parts, it is in fact only 2: on the outside, a black ring that represents all other traditional arts and the importance of showing respect, as we are all on a common journey.

And in the center, at our core, a solid black circle so students never forget that what we do is different.

Name, crests, logos

The Pine Lake Shibu uses a stylized calligraphy as well as the crest from the Onaga Dojo. The calligraphy is intended not only to be read as the Japanese Kanji for "Shinjinbukan" but also represents a strong and bold stroke, while still being very fluid and interconnected, both hallmarks of Onaga sensei's Ti. Most importantly, it has a very clear vertical stroke that runs from top to bottom. This is to remind us of the importance of the "Ti" that runs through our Karate, and that Onaga sensei has always said, "Ti is the backbone of a Tijigaya." Tijigaya is the Okinawa term used for a person who possesses the skill, knowledge, and understanding of Ti.

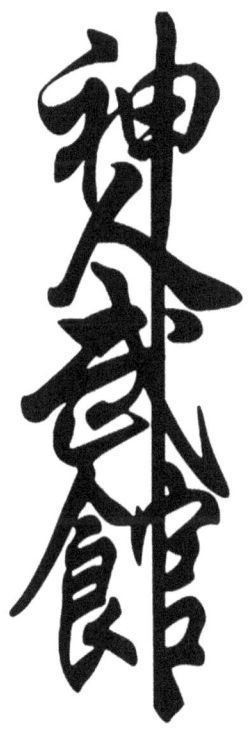

The right to wear either the crest or the calligraphy is not granted or extended in a formal event, but when given, is usually considered a sign of the student's acceptance into the Dojo. I wasn't offered the ability to wear the Onaga Dojo Keikogi until my second year in the Dojo.

Although the Pine Lake Dojo has no hard and fast rule about when a student will receive the crest, calligraphy, and arm patches, it's customary that a student might wait 6-12 months.

It's important to note that the calligraphy is not "hand written," "brushed," or "typed" and would not be understood as natural by native speakers. It is more akin to a logo. In an attempt to convey the "feeling" to someone who does not read Kanji, I created a similar logo in western script in the hopes of providing insight into how the Japanese logo might feel to someone who reads Kanji.

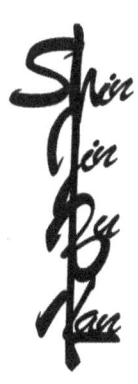

小林流空手道

"Shorin-ryu Karate Do" arm patch, worn with the crest on the arm.

神人武館小林流

"Shinjinbukan Shorin-ryu" arm patch, worn with the crest on the chest.

115

Keikogi

Often referred to simply as "Gi" in English or sometimes "Kimono" in other languages, these terms are technically incorrect. Gi (着) means clothes or garment and wouldn't usually be used on its own in the context of Karate. A Kimono is a formal Japanese garment. Terms like Karategi, Keikogi, and Dogi are all acceptable and interchangeably used in Japanese Dojo.

Although there is neither a need to wear a Keikogi when training, nor a "correct" style of Dogi, we tend to wear our Karategi either with short or long trousers and the jacket sleeves cropped at the elbows.

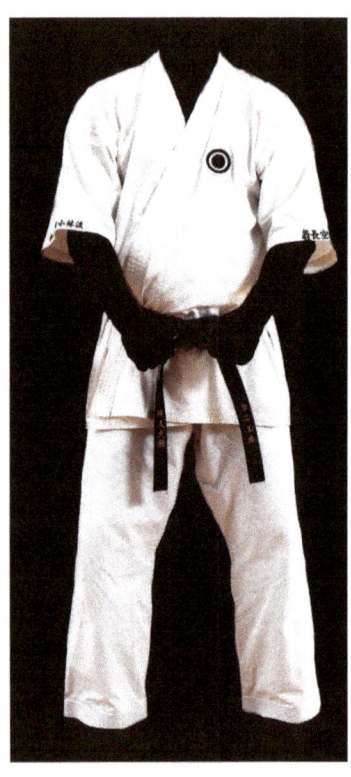

The first Onaga Karate Dojo Keikogi had the crest on the left chest with the Kanji "Onaga Karate Dojo" on the left sleeve. At the turn of the millennium, when the Dojo formally started using the name Shinjinbukan, that Kanji was added to the right sleeve as seen here.

The Obi (帯, belt) is embroidered in yellow (gold) stitching "Shinjinbukan" on one end, worn to right side and the student's name either in Kanji or Katakana on the left.

The sleeves of the Keikogi are cut above the elbows to allow the teacher to see the arm position when training.

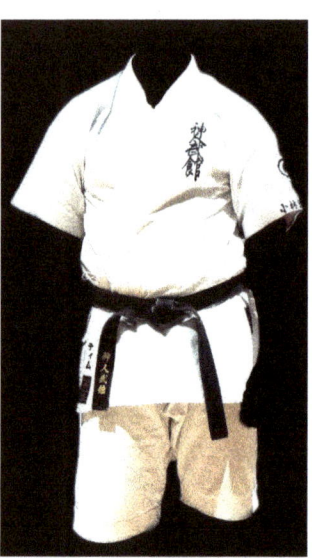

The Pine Lake Shibu also uses the stylized calligraphy, so when that is embroidered on the chest, the crest is placed on the arm. Below the crest one will usually find the Kanji for "Shorin-ryu Karate Do."

There is also an option to place the Dojo name on the left sleeve and the Kanji for "Shinjinbukan Karate Do" on the right, which is the way most students at the Hombu Dojo had it in recent years.

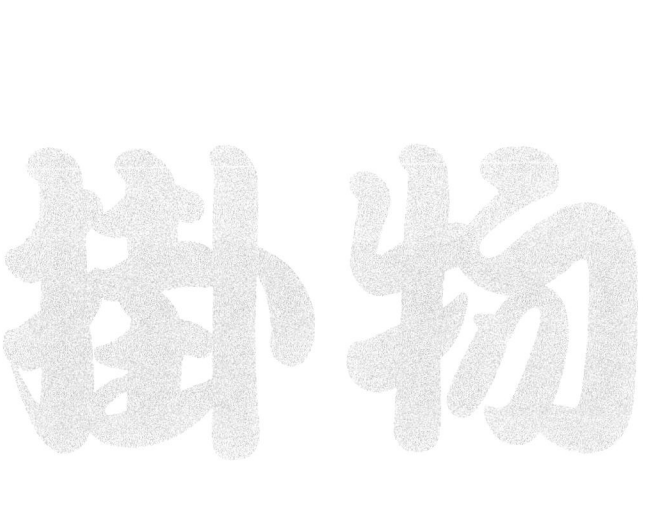
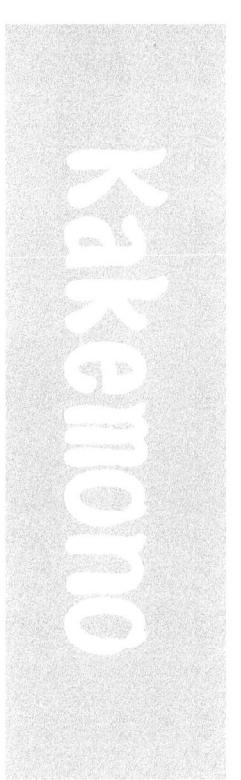

Kakemono (掛物, hanging scrolls), are a traditional part of most Dojo, but they are far more than simple decoration. While most western Dojo might have posters on the walls, a traditional Dojo will usually have a few very specific items, such as the Dojo Kun (道場訓) and Nafudakake (名札掛け) at a minimum. The Dojo Kun are the precepts of the style or school and the Nafuda is the official membership and rank board.

Along with the Dojo Kun and Nafuda, I have several pieces of calligraphy on my walls, mostly items gifted to the Dojo, as well as my most recent rank and teacher's license issued by my sensei.

I'm often asked what they all mean, and, in retrospect, it makes sense that people would want to know. So, here are the items that are currently in my Dojo and their meanings. I share these not because they are particularly great art, although some are, but because of what each piece means to me and my Dojo.

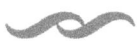

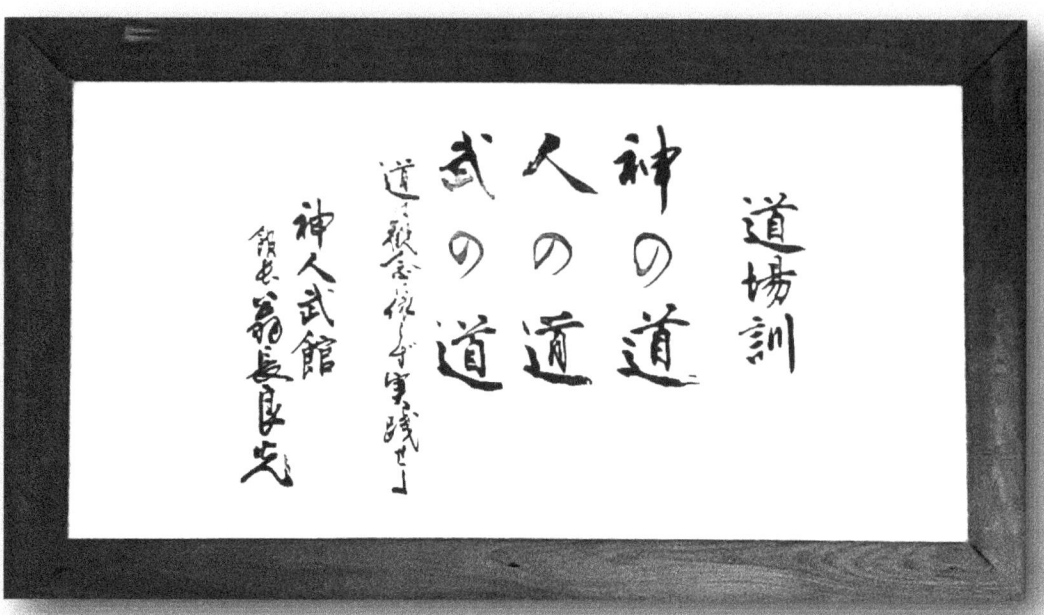

Dojo Kun Dojo affirmation
Kami no Michi The spiritual way
Hito no Michi The human (civil) way
Bu no Michi The martial way
Michi wa kannen ni yorazu jissen seyo The way is attained through practice, not contemplation.

The text is Onaga sensei's Dojo creed/precepts. The brushwork was commissioned in 1990 and brushed by a calligrapher in Tokyo. The work is unsigned because it bears Onaga sensei's name on the lefthand corner, as it is his words and not those of the artist. I was given a copy by sensei in 1992. The alternate reading for Kami and Hito are Shin and Jin respectively. When read from right to left, as intended, it reads Shin, Jin, Bu forming the name of the Dojo, Shinjinbukan.

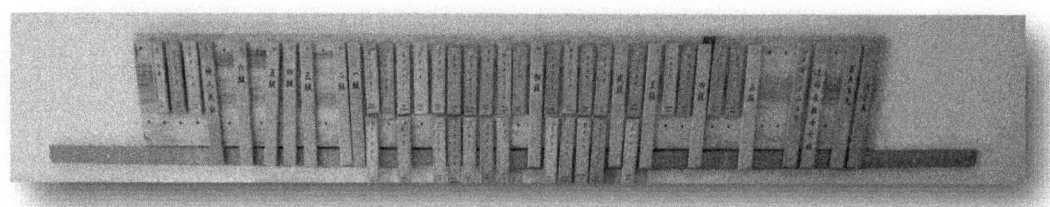

The Nafuda Kake at my Dojo. I keep the names of all students that have received rank (Shodan and higher) from me on the Nafuda. Some schools only keep the names of students actively training at that specific branch Dojo and routinely purge name plates.

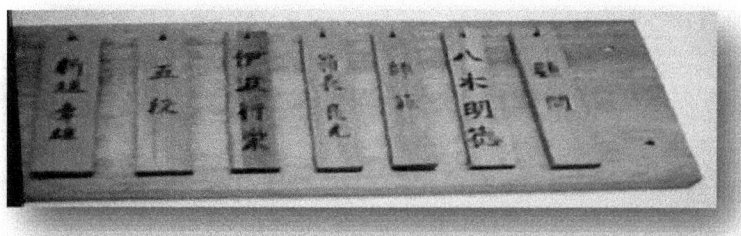

Here is the senior most position of the Nafuda at the Onaga Karate Dojo when I first was permitted to train. It names Yagi Meitoku as the Komon (advisor) for the school, to the right of Onaga sensei, followed by Iha Koei sensei to his left.

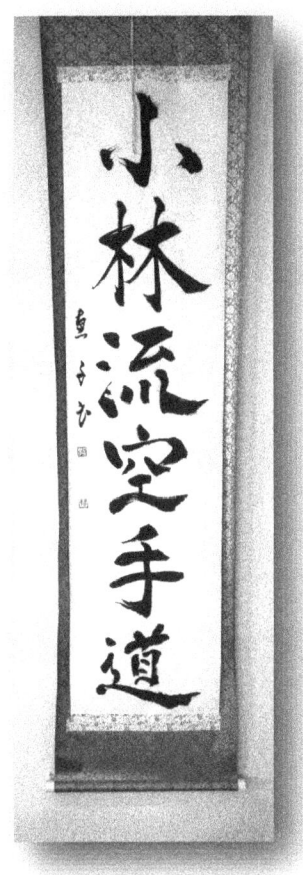

Shorin-ryu Karate Do

Gift from the Kumon Juku Teachers Association in Okinawa, 1991. Brushed by one of the association members.

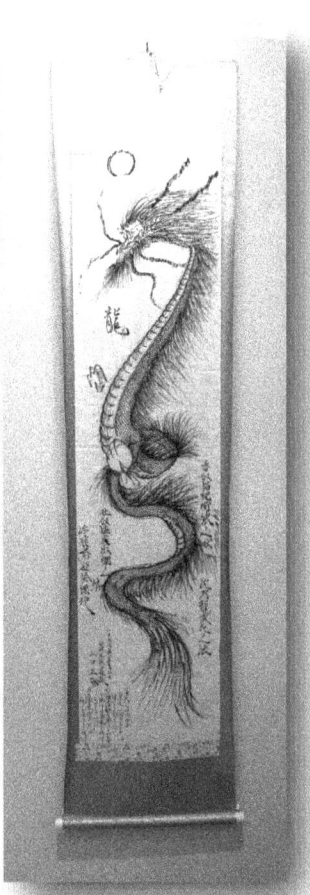

Brushed and gifted to me by Yamaguchi Masahiro Shihan, Matsumura Seito Shorin-ryu.

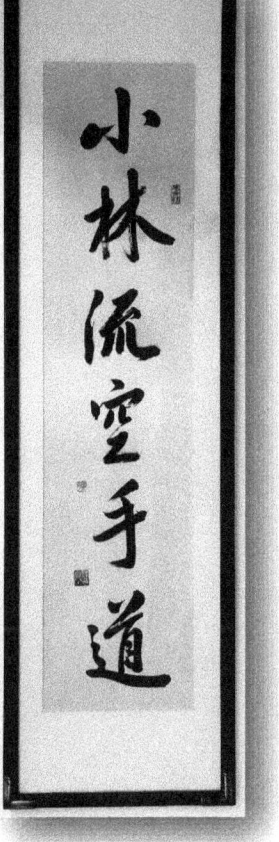

Shorin-ryu Karate Do

Gift from Nikolaos Kontogiannis sifu, head instructor of Yee Yung Tong, Vancouver, Canda, 1996.

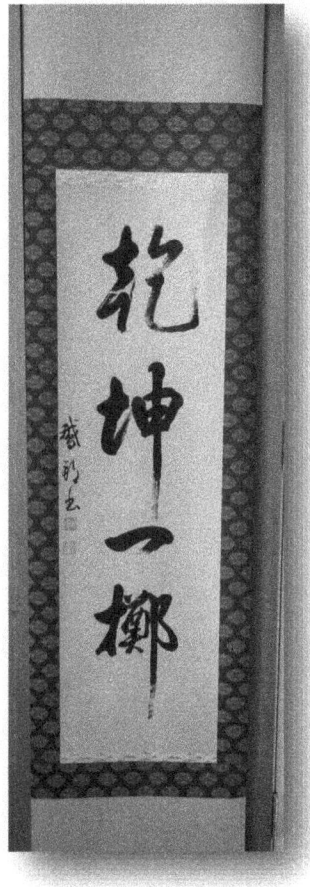

Ken Kon Itteki

"To be fully committed" a gift from Minato Kisaburo, Tokyo, 2013.

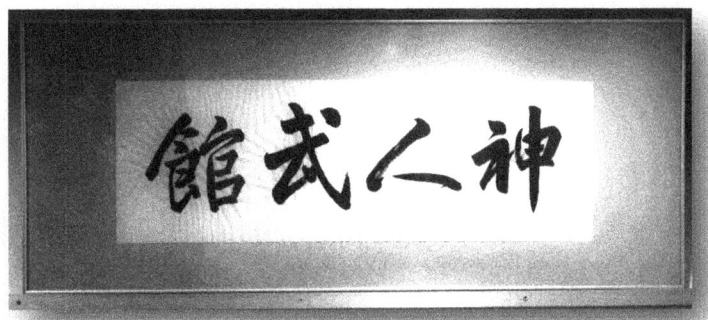

Shinjinbukan

A gift brushed by Ho Ip Sau Fong (1917-2019) my wife's great-aunt. Vancouver, Canada, 2010.

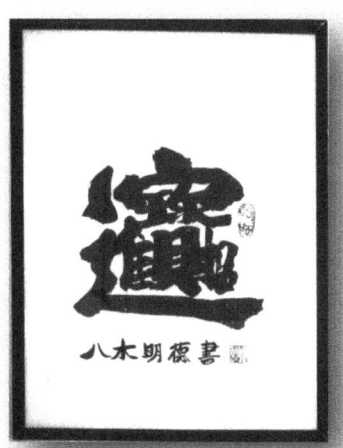

A "poem" brushed by Yagi Meitoku
10th Dan, Meibukan Goju-ryu.
Presented to me by him in 1991.

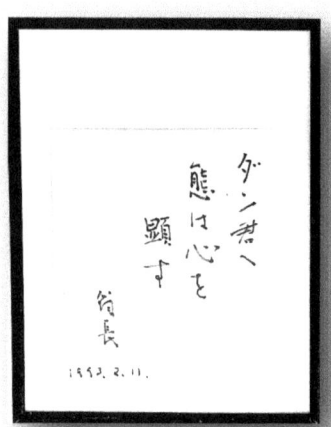

Dan kun e Tai wa kokoro o arawasu

"For Dan, your attitude/behavior reveals your heart"
Written for me by Onaga Yoshimitsu sensei, 1993.

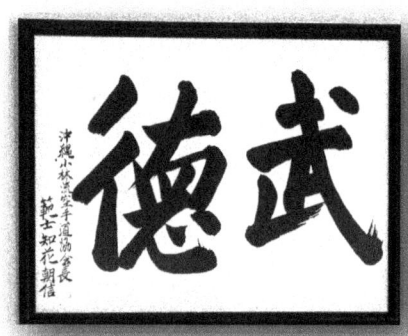

Butoku

"Martial Virtue"
Brushed by Chibana Choshin sensei, copy gifted to me by Ernesto Estrada (Kyoshi), 1999.

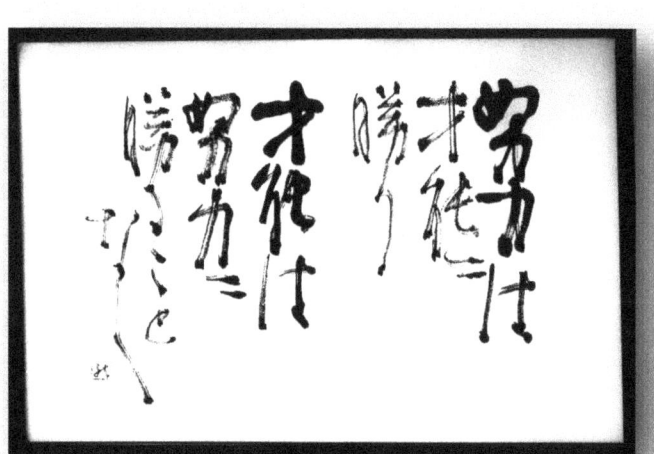

Doryoku wa sainou ni masari   sainou wa doryoku ni masaru koto nashi

"Hard work beats talent when talent fails to work hard"
Brushed by Noriko Thygessen, commissioned in 2018.

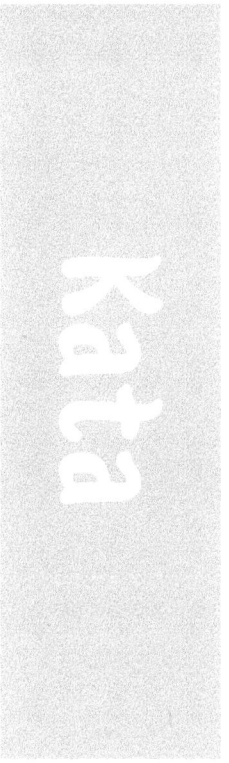

Kata

Kata (型) is many things. The easiest and most basic way to understand it is as a syllabus of ideas and techniques, used to cultivate muscle memory. It is also a very practical tool to use as a yardstick to measure the mechanical aspects of doing a technique; direction, height, size, etc.… But the most important use of Kata is as a list of ideas committed to memory from which to select when practicing in front of a Machiwara or partner. Kata is not the goal. One will often hear people say that Kata is the essence of Karate. At the Onaga Dojo, Kata was always considered a tool to be used, polished, sharpened, and strengthened in order to improve our Karate.

Kata changes as both the student's and teacher's understanding evolves, or devolves in some cases. If anyone ever says they are doing or teaching the "original" version of a Kata, either they don't know better or they assume the listener doesn't. Kata is one gateway to learning Ti, and, as such, just like Ti is personal and specific to a teacher, as in Onaga no Ti, so is Kata. One can say they do the Kata as done or taught by a teacher you've had direct contact with, and that's about all that can be said about Kata.

Kata

Kata names are a source of much debate and are fairly arbitrary. Teachers reused names and changed forms to be unrecognizable, but often maintained the "old name." The application of Kanji was more political or aspirational than related to the actual Kata. It is for this reason that Kata names are often written in phonetics, Katakana, rather than Kanji. This attributes no meaning to the name and is simply the sound of the words, more like a proper name than a description with meaning. For this list, I have simply avoided the problem and used the common Romaji.

It's important to note that although there are many wrong ways to do Kata, there is no single "right way." It depends on the student's Busai (武歳), martial age - skill level and understanding. As a result, Kata very often have 3, 4, or more versions that students progress through, eventually reaching the appropriate level for them.

Kihon Gata: Basic form. There are 4 Kihon Gata sets that we do, each with 3 to 7 sections per Kata. Many Shorin-ryu schools do 3 Kihon Gata. They are most often attributed to Chibana Choshin sensei (1885-1969). We've grouped these 3 sets to make what we refer to as the first basic form, Dai Ichi Kihon Gata. Each of the Kihon Gata are sets of variations on a particular exercise. Dai Ichi Kihon Gata is done in Shizentai going forward and Neko Ashi and Uke Ashi when retreating. Dai Ni Kihon Gata (second basic form) was created by Onaga sensei and is a series consisting of 7 sections, each with a different block followed by Mae Geri and Tsuki, each section done in Zenkutsu Dachi, both forward and retreating in a straight line. Dai San Kihon Gata and Dai Yon Kihon Gata are done in Jigotai and Shiko Dachi respectively, based on exercises attributed to Higa Yuchoku (1919 –1994) and standardized by Onaga sensei. Dai San consists of 3 sections and Dai Yon of 4 sections. Dai San Kihon is done using Sankaku Tenshin footwork, while Dai Yon is a straight line.

All the Kihon Gata have no set count; you advance until you've had enough, you've run out of room, or are instructed to retreat.

Pinan Gata: A series of 5 Kata. Attributed to Itosu Anko sensei (1831-1915). They are said to be derived from an existing version of a more complex Kata at the time, as a way to introduce Karate into the Okinawa school system's physical education curriculum. These are numbered one through five: Pinan Shodan, Nidan, Sandan, Yondan, Godan.

Kata

Naihanchi Gata: A series of 3 Kata, Naihanchi Shodan, Nidan, Sandan. These are considered to be the "yardstick" we use for measuring/checking the rest of our Karate. These Kata are where students will learn how to generate power from the hip, Kushijike, as well as proper breathing, posture, balance, and Chinkuchi. Naihanchi are usually done in a straight line, with the stance feet shoulder width apart pointing forward, or slightly inwards; this position is referred to as Naihanchi Dachi.

Jion Gata: This Kata introduces a series of new ideas about extending and stretching the techniques. It is where we see the longest Zenkutsu Dachi we do, as well as introduces the nearly ubiquitous circular *en garde* positions of the Onaga Dojo.

Chinto Gata: An intermediate level Kata, characterized by its use of Tsuru Ashi Dachi, crane leg stance. The other notable technique, mostly because we tend not to show it, is the Nidan Mae Tobi Geri, two-level jumping front kick. It is commonly done as two Mae Geri.

Useishin Gata: Often called Gojushiho in Japanese, introduces several new concepts and targets not seen in previous Kata. The change of directions, the intentional leaning into and away from the opponent, as well as the deliberate change in height, make it feel different from most other Kata. This Kata was not commonly done at the Onaga Dojo.

Note: I've learned several versions of this Kata over the years of training, in Argentina as well as on Okinawa. The version we do is the one I learned directly from Onaga sensei and the version I was responsible for teaching at the Hombu Dojo on occasion.

Unsu Gata: Perhaps the least common and most misunderstood Kata practiced at the Onaga Dojo. There are countless Kata in other lineages and styles that use the name Unsu that have nothing to do with this Kata. There are a few schools on Okinawa whose Unsu bears a resemblance and we can see the common lineage. What makes this version of Unsu so different is not the Embusen but the body mechanics. It is Onaga sensei's contention that a student should not learn Unsu until they have managed to internalize the Passai Kata. The reason is that the body mechanics of Unsu are completely contrary to how power is generated in Passai, and trying to learn both at the same time simply doesn't work.

Note: I learned Unsu from Iha Koei sensei 9th Dan Kyudokan Shorin-ryu. Since this was Iha sensei's trademark Kata, Onaga sensei asked him to teach it to his daughter and me in the mid-90s.

Kata

Sochin Gata and **Seisan Gata**: A pair of Kata that are similar in the body mechanics and fighting principles. These Kata were not trained at the Onaga Dojo. I have learned several versions of these Kata over the years and worked to introduce the concepts that are common across other forms in the Shinjinbukan to the way I train these Kata.

Note: Although Onaga sensei didn't ever teach these, I have reviewed them with sensei and have received guidance from him on both. An interesting note about Seisan, and the reason I have incorporated it into my teaching, is that this is the only Kata that is found across all the major styles of Karate on Okinawa.

Jitte Gata: This Kata was not taught or trained at the Onaga Dojo. It has a few unique movements and change of directions. The most notable move comes near the end of the Kata with Sagurite no Kamae done with a closed fist.

Note: Like most of the Kata that I practice and teach that were not part of the Onaga Dojo curriculum, I have learned multiple versions over the years and settled on a form that feels like and incorporates the fundamentals of the Kata we train.

Passai Gata: There are two, Passai no Sho (小) and Passai no Dai (大). Unfortunately, this naming convention has resulted in a lot of confusion. Sho is often translated to mean "small" and Dai "big." The movements of Passai no Sho are typically larger, more open movements, while Passai no Dai tend to be smaller, inside fighting ideas. As the students grow in knowledge and skill, the techniques get smaller and more precise. So rather than thinking about these as small and large, it is better to understand these as "lesser" and "greater" Passai, where the name denotes the skill level required. An interesting trait of the Passai Kata is that they introduce a series of new fighting strategies not seen in other forms. They focus on baiting the opponent, controlling the perceived openings in one's own defense, and manipulating the attacker's instincts to one's advantage.

Note: Of all the Kata Onaga sensei learned and taught, Passai is where he has spent the greatest amount of time and effort and as a result, these Kata are what we consider to be the hallmark of Shinjinbukan Kata.

Kusanku Gata: This set of two Kata are also named using the Sho and Dai taxonomy and, like Passai, should be understood as the "lesser" and "greater" Kusanku Kata. Many Shorin-ryu schools consider Kusanku no Dai to be the most advanced Kata, but that is a relatively modern idea. Kata are as advanced, deep, or shallow, as the practitioner's understanding. Kusanku Kata tend to focus primarily on evading, slipping past techniques and inside the guard.

The Kata taught at the Onaga Dojo were primarily the list of Kata that sensei directly attributed to Chibana Chosin sensei: Pinan Gata, Naihanchi Gata, Jion, Chinto, Passai Sho/Dai, Kusanku Sho/Dai. Other Kata were both taught and practiced but it was always understood they were extracurricular.

Rank

Rank is probably the single most misunderstood part of Karate. What rank means and what it represents tend to be much more an expression of the student-teacher relationship and the person's place and role within the Dojo, than anything else. This is certainly true for the senior ranks. Shodan (初段, first degree) through to Yondan (四段, fourth degree) have more emphasis on specific technical requirements in our Dojo and, as a result, are probably more clearly defined.

There are several types of rank, but most important, if any rank can be said to be important, is Shodan, which represents a basic level of competency and admittance into the Dojo, as a formal student. Some schools make a distinction between Dojo rank and that issued by an association. There is only one type of rank in our Dojo: that which is issued by the teacher (Dojocho or Shihan) to a direct student.

Belts and rank are complicated. They are not at all the point of learning and doing Karate, and yet most of us have received rank, have strived to attain it, and some of us have issued rank. There is no governing body that sets standards or expectations for each rank. As a result, rank has little meaning without the context of who issued it, when, and to whom. What rank means and the value it represents are essentially "in the eye of the beholder."

In the Shinjinbukan, the order of the Kata loosely correlates to the student's rank, and so they are listed here together. There is no fixed order, since each student learns at their own pace and in their own way. It is expected that students should know all the Kata by the rank of Nidan. This is a general rule and does not always apply. It happens on occasion that a students may not know or do all the Kata by Nidan, but it is never the case that a student is required to wait for a particular rank to learn a particular Kata.

Rank aside, we typically spend the first 12-24 months working on Naihanchi Shodan, nearly exclusively when training Kata. It's possible that other Kata are introduced but less likely that they are checked or corrected in much detail. The focus is on body mechanics, posture, breathing, and power via Naihanchi.

段位 Rank

Kata	Rank	
Dai ichi Kihon Gata	10級 (Jukyu)	
Naihanchi Shodan Gata	9級 (Kukyu)	
Pinan Nidan Gata	8級 (Hachikyu)	
Dai ni Kihon Gata	7級 (Nanakyu)	
Pinan Shodan Gata	6級 (Rokyu)	
Pinan Sandan Gata / Naihanchi Nidan Gata	5級 (Gokyu)	
Pinan Yondan Gata / Pinan Godan Gata / Naihanchi Sandan Gata	4級 (Yonkyu)	

Iro Obi, color belts, usually children's belts. Other colors were also used for children at the Onaga Dojo when children's classes were offered.

Jion Gata / Dai San Kihon Gata	3級 (Sankyu)
Dai Yon Kihon Gata	2級 (Nikyu)
Chinto Gata / Passai No sho Gata	1級 (Ikkyu)

Beginner adult students (16 years or older) typically only have white or brown belts before reaching black belts. Stripes may be used starting from 5th kyu which is typically the first rank awarded to adults.

| Jitte Gata / Seisan Gata / Sochin Gata / Kusanku No sho Gata / Unsu Gata | 1段 (Shodan) |

Kuro Obi, black belt

Not all Kata listed are taught or trained today at the Hombu Dojo. This list of Kata is presented here in the order in which they are typically taught in my Dojo.

| Useishin Gata / Passai No dai Gata / Kusanku No dai Gata | 2段 (Nidan) |

All Kata are required by Nidan, in accordance to the rank requirements guidelines.

Rank

無段者 Mudansha Rank (all ranks below Shodan)

All rank below Shodan will be issued by the Shibu Dojo (支部道場, branch Dojo). The decision of when to promote a student through the ranks below Shodan will be at the discretion of the Shibucho (支部長, branch manager).

Each Shibucho has the authority and discretion to structure the ranks below black belt as deemed appropriate in his/her region.

有段者 Yudansha ranks (black belt ranks)

Ranks of Shodan, Nidan, and Sandan may be awarded at the discretion of a Shibucho who holds a minimum rank of Yondan.

Minimum Grading Requirements

The grading requirements are a guideline. The ultimate decision for awarding or requesting rank lies with the Shibucho responsible for the Dojo.

Shodan 初段

- ☐ Yobi Undo
- ☐ Reigi Saho
- ☐ Tsuki
- ☐ Tachi Machiwara
- ☐ Keri
- ☐ Sagi Machiwara
- ☐ Tachi Kata
- ☐ Tenshin
- ☐ Kigu Undo
- ☐ Hojo Undo
- ☐ Seiri Undo

Nidan 弐段

All Kata in order

Sandan 三段

A total of 30 pair techniques, including 10 Iri Kumi techniques

Yondan 四段

Free Tenshin
Atifa in both Tsuki and Keri

Rank

Godan 五段

Must be running an active Dojo, must possess the ability to teach the entire Shinjinbukan syllabus.

Rokudan 六段

The ability to do more than 30 Iri Kumi from each of the 3 Kakie positions, as well as all the Machiwara technique, Tsuki, Keri, Tenshin, and all the Kata

Nanadan 七段

Minimum of 5 years after Rokudan and at least 40 years of age.

Hachidan 八段

Minimum of 5 years after Nanadan. You have been recognized beyond any doubt to have a distinguished character and have been recognized for your Busai in Ryukyu no Karate Bushi. Note: there will be no more than 1 Hachidan per country outside of Okinawa.

Kyudan 九段

As a Kyudan, you possess the entire knowledge of the Shinjinbukan, and the ability to do it. You will also be the director of the international representatives and will promote and enforce the Shinjinbukan rules, philosophy and teachings

Judan 十段

In all practical terms, there will be no Judan in the Shinjinbukan. Judan will only be given as an honorary rank upon the death of an active Kyudan, or if a Kyudan reaches the age of 80 years and is still an active Shihan.

Teaching License (instructor rank)

Often you will see an instructor, or senior students in other Dojo, wearing red and white striped belts, or solid red belts. These are a standard practice in Judo and typically denote ranks of 6th Dan or higher. Some schools in Okinawa today also use these red belts and often conflate the Dan ranks with instructor ranks. As a result, one will often see someone promoted to fifth or sixth Dan receive a red and white belt and the title of Renshi. There are no red or red-striped belts in the Shinjinbukan.

Dan ranks should be understood in relation to the student's ability and place in the Dojo, and not as a statement of their ability to teach and produce students.

Even when red belts are not used, it is not uncommon for specific Dan ranks to be automatically mapped to instructor ranks. In our Dojo, this is not the case. Instructor ranks Renshi (錬士), Kyoshi (教士), Hanshi (範士) are independent from black belt ranks. There is a correlation since it's unlikely that someone could obtain an instructor rank and not have attained a significant Dan rank. Dan ranks are "necessary but not sufficient." Having a fifth Dan does not make you a qualified teacher. The other "rank" often used and rarely understood is Shihan (師範) which is

段位 Rank

actually not a rank or title that is ever awarded per se, but rather a way to express a teacher's role within the Dojo structure. The easiest way to think about this is the common usage of "sensei" that we all understand to mean teacher. Nobody hands out "sensei" certificates, or at least they shouldn't. What makes someone a teacher is that they have students. That is the definition of a teacher. It is not a statement or endorsement of their ability to teach, but rather a recognition of the facts. There is no rank requirement; it is the students that make the teacher, and by students using the term "sensei", they have entered into a student-teacher relationship. The term Shihan is similar. It is an acknowledgement that a teacher is a teacher of teachers. More simply put, their students also teach. If this were put in the form of a family tree, a grandparent by definition has grandchildren, a Shihan by definition has students who teach a third generation of students.

Returning to the titles and ranks issued for instructors, Renshi, Kyoshi, and Hanshi are denoted by using yellow/gold stripes on a black belt, as well as the issuance of a certificate. One, two, and three stripes, respectively, may be placed on one or both ends of a black belt.

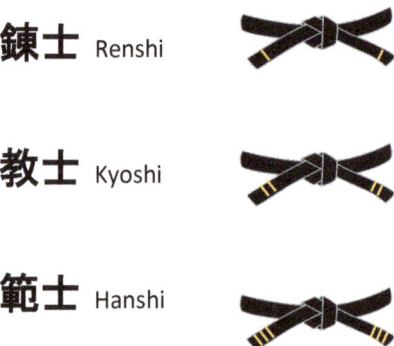

Nafuda or Nafudakake (名札掛け), meaning name plate, or perhaps better stated as name plate rack, is probably the best way to understand a student's place in the Dojo and the rank that has been awarded to them. The Nafuda will have the names of the students who are in good standing organized by rank. It will often have the name plate of the head of the Dojo and sometimes the name plate of the authority under which the rank was issued, so you will find students, the teacher, the head of the style on the "rank board" and sometimes the name of a Komon, or advisors (顧問).

Rank Certificates

証明

Shoumei (証明), meaning "to prove," is the paper manifestation of the teacher reading (or saying) out loud that a student has attained a certain rank. We usually say "certificate," but it's commonly understood that rank is awarded when the teacher reads the words out loud. Even when it's been just sensei and me alone in the room, he would read it out loud as he awarded the rank and handed me the certificate. Rank certificates are nothing more than a letter or receipt stating that a student has been recognized as having achieved a specific rank by whoever's signature is on the certificate. In fact, some Japanese arts issue scrolls, rather than flat paper certificates, but essentially it is just a letter. There is no "official" style or type of certificate. They have changed over the years and tend to either follow the latest "fashion" or are designed to appeal to the esthetics of the person whose signature it bears.

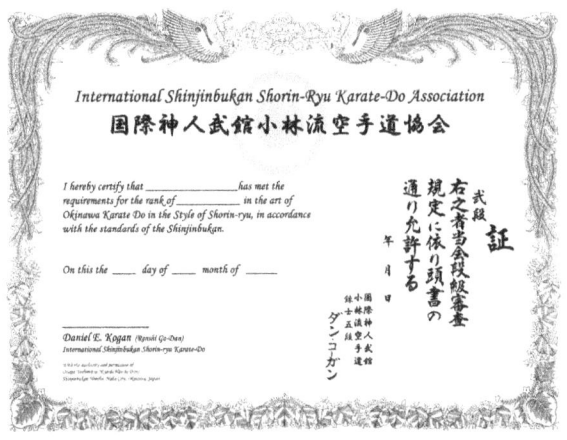

This is what the early certificates issued from 1993 through to 2011 at my Dojo looked like. These included the common gold frame often seen in Japanese certificates. It also includes a copy of the Japanese text used on the Hombu Dojo rank certificates at the time, and an English language text.

Starting in 2012, certificates issued from the Pine Lake Shibu are as seen here.

The text is still the original text from the early Onaga Karate Dojo, although formatted differently and now includes the Pine Lake Shibu stylized calligraphy. The outer frame was dropped to bring it more in line with the esthetics of the certificates issued at the Hombu Dojo.

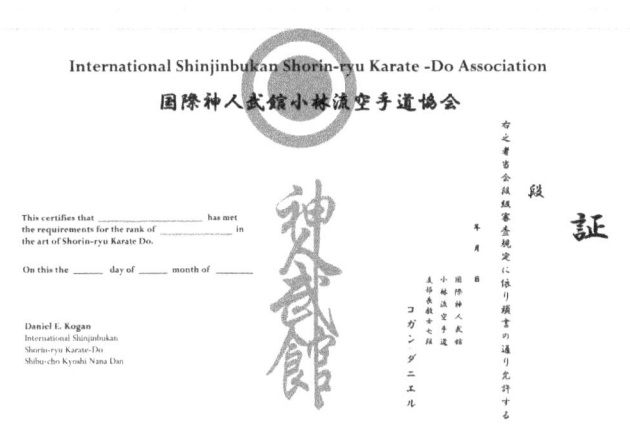

証明 Rank Certificates

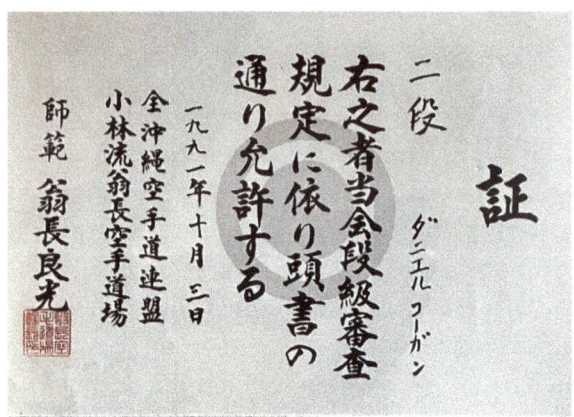

A certificate from the Onaga Karate Dojo, issued by sensei in 1991. It makes no use of the name "Shinjinbukan." It identifies the Dojo as a member of the Zen Okinawa Karate Do Renmei (All Okinawa Karate Do Federation), and uses the name Shorin-ryu Onaga Karate Dojo.

Some time around the turn of the millennium was when Onaga sensei changed the formal name of his Dojo to Shinjinbukan, and the certificates issued changed to those seen here.

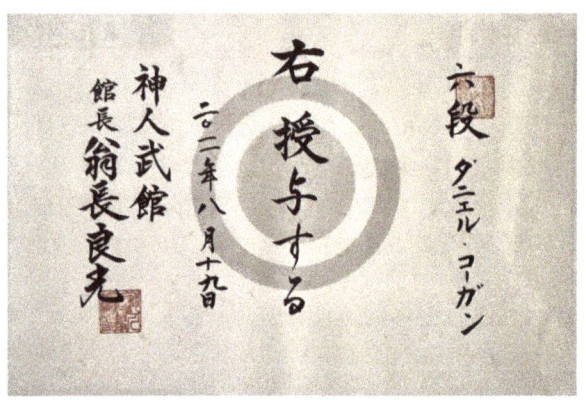 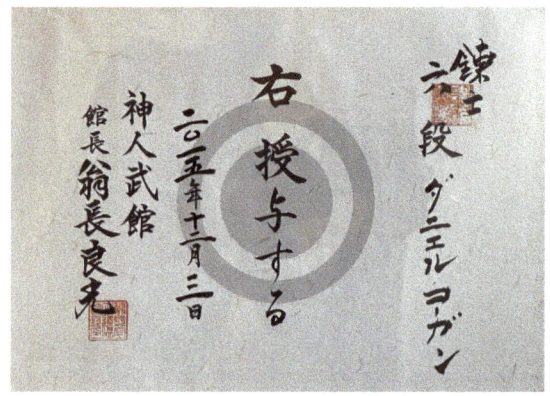

It's important to note a few other changes. The text has been reduced to a very simple statement that translates close to "conferred, bestowed, granted" and includes the name, rank of the recipient to the right, as well as the date, title, and name of the authority issuing the certificate to the left. When a teaching license is awarded, it is explicitly indicated on the certificate as seen in the second Rokudan certificate above with the added "Renshi" or the "Kyoshi" in the Nanadan certificate below.

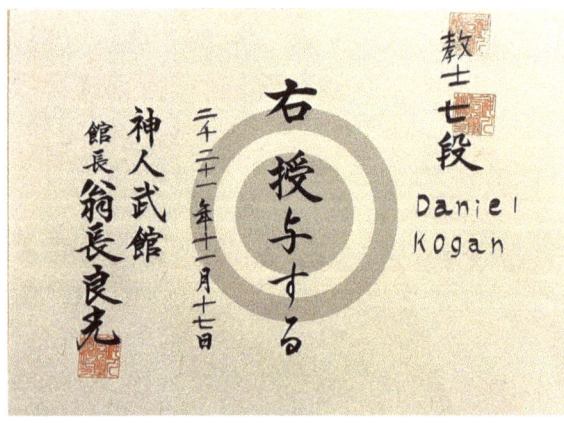

Certificates have usually been filled out by the acting Dojo secretary, although not always, some were penned by Onaga sensei while others simply received his Hanko (seal) after being completed by the Dojo secretary.

As a result you can see that the way names are presented has changed over the years.

Dojo Genealogy

小林流 Shorin-ryu

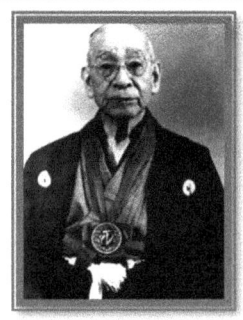

Chibana Choshin (1885 - 1969)

剛柔流 Goju-ryu

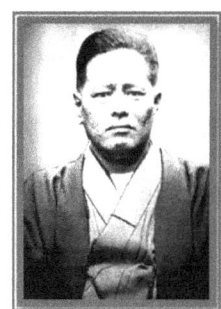

Miyagi Chojun (1888 - 1953)

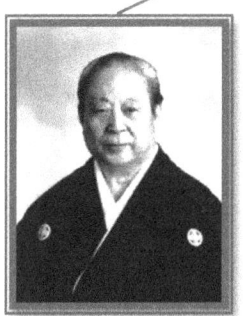

Miyahira Katsuya (1918 - 2010)

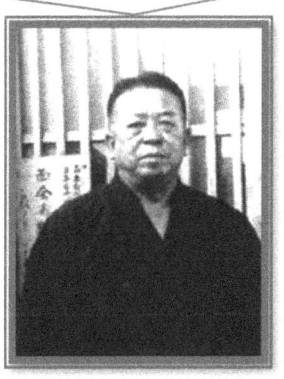

Higa Yuchoku (1910 - 1994)

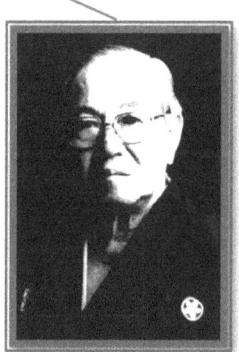

Yagi Meitoku (1912 - 2006)

Advisor (Komon 顧問)

It was under the guidance and with the encouragement of Yagi sensei that the Onaga Dojo opened in 1988.

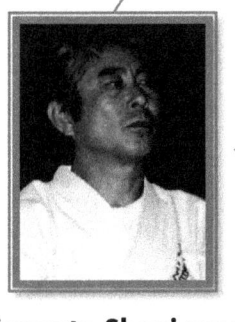

Miyazato Shoei (1935 - 2013)

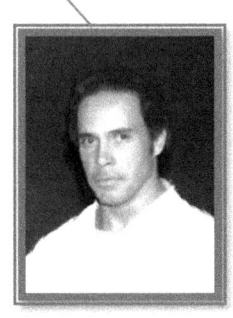

J.J. Brinkmann (1945 - 1989)

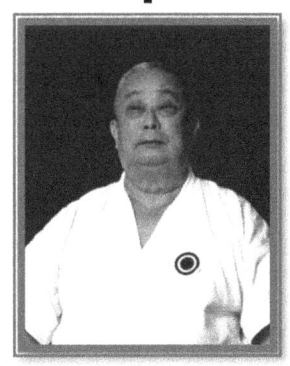

Onaga Yoshimitsu (1938 -)

I first met Onaga sensei in 1988 in Buenos Aires, Argentina, and was accepted into his Dojo and formally as his student in 1989.

My introduction to Shorin-ryu was in Buenos Aires, Argentina, 1986. Brinkmann sensei is responsible for getting me started on my journey.

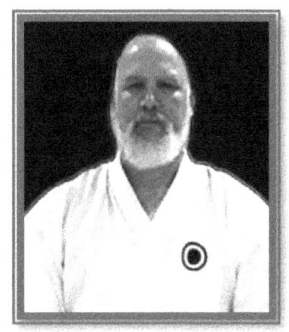

Daniel Kogan (1968 -)

<u>Note</u>: only teachers directly impacting the Karate we train today are listed here.

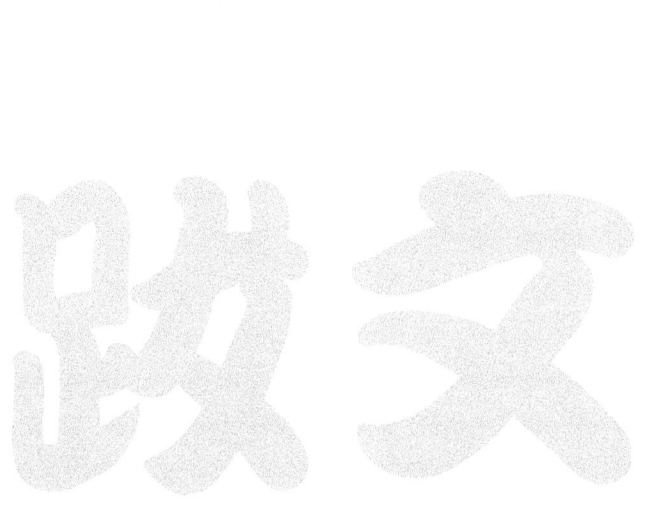
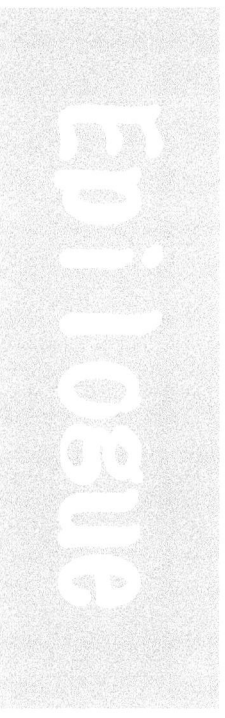

Epilogue

The current volume was intended to be a technical manual for students interested in getting a peek into the training and Dojo culture practiced at the Matsu Mizumi Shibu Dojo (Pine Lake Branch Dojo) of the Shinjinbukan.

Although the terms Karate and Ti might appear to have been used interchangeably throughout this book, the reader should understand that Onaga sensei makes a clear and purposeful distinction between the two.

When I first became Onaga sensei's student, I joined the "Onaga **<u>Karate</u>** Dojo", prior to which I had done sports Karate for a decade in Canada and had had a taste of Okinawan Karate while living in South America in 1987, but it was the small taste of Onaga sensei's Karate in Buenos Aires in 1989 that motivated me to venture, uninvited, to the other side of the globe, where I "earned" my way into the Dojo. It was then, after Onaga sensei allowed me to join his Karate Dojo and, despite years of prior training, that I started my karate journey anew.

I don't recall hearing sensei use the term "Ti" for the first few years that I trained at the Dojo and, if he had used it, I certainly didn't understand what it meant. Which is an important lesson in and of itself. While I was learning and doing Karate, much of it I absorbed by watching and copying, or at least I thought as much, but the lack of language skills was a severely limiting factor. If I didn't manage to get some Japanese language under my belt, no matter how rudimentary, the interactions with people and, therefore, the learning I'd experience would never reach the depth and nuance that I sought and which sensei demanded

During one class, after several years together, in an attempt to have me grasp what he was explaining, I recall sensei saying, "Kore Wa Karate Jania, Korre Wa Ti. Ti Wa Chie" (これは空手じゃない。これは手。手は知恵。), This is not karate. This is Ti. Ti is wisdom.

With the help of a dictionary, I got the meaning of the phrase but did not realize at the time how profound and impactful this simple statement would become in my training, my life, my relationship with sensei and in the lives of my students.

Over thirty years later, the term Ti has become rather trendy amongst Karate exponents, around the world, particularly those in the realm of cyberspace. Ti is often said to be an arcane term for Karate, or proclaimed to be "the original" native fighting art of the Ryukyuan archipelago. Although not completely incorrect, that way of thinking about Ti suggests that it is like a style or an art form which includes, or excludes, certain techniques and ideas. One might ask, is a jumping-spinning hook kick Ti? Probably not, but not for the reasons most would assume. It is true that the jumping-spinning hook kick is not in any of the Kata we train and, for many, that method of determination defines the parameters for what constitutes allowable techniques under the banner of what is considered Ti. However, the fact that this technique does not appear in Kata is not the issue, as learning Ti is not necessarily about Kata. I would argue that a jumping-spinning hook kick isn't Ti because it violates many of the basic tenets of what we consider appropriate, effective, and efficient technique upon which one would risk one's life. Understanding and accepting that real fighting always and inevitably entails a significant level of risk, turning one's back to the opponent while standing on one leg, or even worse while jumping in the air, and attempting to hit one's opponent in the head violates so many core principles that it would never be viewed as the best option when looking through the lens of Ti. That's not to say one couldn't score a point in a controlled situation with a referee to stop the bout when things go wrong, or that one might even, on a rare occasion, connect the heel with an opponent's jaw or back of the head with varying results. But when one is gambling with one's life, those kinds of odds are far too risky. This type of understanding and way of thinking about techniques, body mechanics, and inherent real-world risks are examples of the "wisdom" Onaga sensei talks about when he says, Ti wa Chie. Ti is always about the *best* option, the one that allows a smaller and weaker person to not be beaten by a larger, stronger assailant. When looking through the lens of Ti, a jumping-spinning anything is unlikely, if ever, going to meet this standard.

Shinmen Musashi, better known as Miyamoto Musashi, in his 17th century treatise on swordsmanship, *The Book of Five Rings*, used the term Heiho (兵法) commonly translated as "strategy". It is a worldview, a way of understanding technique, human behavior, one's role in combat, when to engage and when to avoid conflict, one's place in the Dojo, and a way of understanding one's role in society. Bearing Musashi's teachings in mind, observing and copying movements will never unlock a teacher's ideas and understanding for a student, nor will miming movements help one see that each teacher will have slightly different, sometimes radically different, understandings to convey. What matters most is understanding that each teacher's lived experiences become the defining elements of their particular Ti, or Heiho.

Wisdom is the ability to make decisions based on one's lived experiences and deep understandings of one's chosen path. It involves the ability to see situations from multiple perspectives and to anticipate the consequences of one's and another's actions, based on detailed and consistently applied principles. This way of understanding Ti is not about a specific technique, or a particular exercise being included in the canon of an art known as Ti, but about a way of thinking, understanding, and evaluating options and outcomes when one's life depends on it.

With this in mind, I encourage the reader to continue their own journey of learning with the second volume in this set, entitled *Hard Lessons Learned the Hard Way*. *Hard Lessons* goes beyond technical descriptions allowing the reader to walk alongside and glimpse into the lived experiences that have shaped Onaga no Ti and the Karate taught at the Shinjinbukan today. Told through the stories Onaga sensei shared with me about his own journey, and through the experiences we shared together as teacher and student, volume two opens a unique window for the reader to peer into the little known, and often misunderstood, world of Karate, Ti, and life as an Uchi Deshi.

vocabulary

As already discussed in the Preface, this manual is not a language course, but since Karate is primarily an oral tradition, language is important and so a vocabulary list is necessary.

Okinawa Karate Dojo tend to have fewer agreed upon terms than mainland Dojo and typically rely on descriptions rather than labels for techniques; as a result, the same idea may have several "names" depending on the Dojo or instructor. This is often a source of frustration for westerners expecting each technique to have a standardized name.

In the following pages are some terms that should hopefully help, but it's important that this not be considered the definitive meaning, use, or expression, but rather the way these ideas were expressed and taught while I was at the Onaga Dojo.

Because techniques tend to be described rather than named, much of the list is common Japanese language that you might hear in class.

One notable difference between Okinawan Dojo and those in mainland Japan is that in most Okinawan Karate Dojo, a technique is referred to by the direction in which it travels, not where it starts or where it ends.

This is why Uchi Uke is a block moving towards the inside, while Age Uke or Age Jichi are rising block and rising strike, respectively. In other words, when referring to a technique like Soto Uke, outside block, the point of reference is the path the technique travels relative to the person doing the technique. A Soto Uke moves towards the outside. It may never reach there but that is the trajectory when it starts moving.

Similarly, Uchi Uke moves towards the inside of the body. A rising strike or block may never reach the head, but it travels in an upward trajectory and so it is Agi Jichi, rising strike in Okinawan or Age Uke, rising block in Japanese. This makes no claim about where the final resting place of the technique will be. In contrast, many mainland Dojo would say Jodan Tsuki, high strike, and think it synonymous to Agi Jichi; in fact, both do use the same 上 Kanji, which causes confusion for Japanese readers. When read Jodan (上段), it is a noun that should translate to upper level, when read Ageru (上げる) it is a verb, that would translate to rising. In the case of the noun, it implies that the technique ends at the "upper level," the head. But when used as a verb, it simply says that the technique is rising from its initial position. The relative size difference between two people may make it that a Jodan Tsuki for one is a Chudan Tsuki for someone else and yet both were Agi Jichi.

ボキャブラリー　　　Vocabulary

A

age from the verb Ageru, to raise; also pronounced "Agi" in Okinawa.
age tsuki rising strike
age uke rising block (usually with the forearm)
agi jichi rising strike (Oki.)
ago jaw
arigato gozaimashita past tense of "thank you very much" to express gratitude for what has already occurred.
arigato gozaimasu thank you very much
aruki kata walking technique/form
asa geiko morning training. Techniques practiced are usually different from those practiced in the evening or night training. Typically, more technical and less strength and cardio in nature.
ashi leg, foot
ashi no yubi toes
atifa the power and technique to defeat an opponent in a single strike (Oki.)

B

barai sweep, as in a leg sweep, Ashibarai or downward sweeping block, Gedanbarai
bogu protective armor
budo (lit. the martial way) a general term used for "martial arts," written as Bu no Michi in the context of the Shinjinbukan Dojo Kun.
bugeisha martial arts person. This term is the formal term for all who learn Bujutsu.
buki weapons
bunkai application of Kata
busai martial age, an individual's depth of knowledge and understanding of Ti

C

chie wisdom
chiishi one-sided weight used as a training tool, Chi=strength and Ishi=stone
chikara strength, power
chinkuchi natural locking position of the muscles
chudan mid-level, mid-section

D

dai sensei Great/grand teacher; the grand master of a style. In more informal speech, it is also used to refer to a teacher two generations above you, similar to "grandfather" "grand teacher."
dan literally step, used to denote black belt levels
dani the ranking system used in the martial arts and other traditional Japanese arts where skill and proficiency is denoted with Dan ranks.
daruma taiso a stretching and strength building exercise typically done in lotus position which involves rolling on the ground while practicing a controlled breathing pattern. Said to resemble the daruma dolls.
deshi disciple
do (lit. the way) alternative reading is "Michi." It is the equivalent to the Chinese term "Tao" and is written with the same character in Japanese and Chinese.
dogi training uniform
dojo often translated as "school," it is a place dedicated to the learning of an art or way
domo "thanks," used in informal settings both as a greeting as well as to say thank you
don to tai inhale exhale pause

E

embusen the pattern traced on the floor when during a kata
empi elbow
enbu (Embu) demonstration

F

findi changing hands (Oki.)
fui jichi swinging strike, sometimes referred to as "reaching" (Oki.)
fuku shibu subbranch, a dojo which is part of a branch of an organization

Vocabulary

fumi komi stomping kick

furoshiki a large kerchief used as a traditional method of carrying small objects. Often used for one's keikogi by placing the item in the center of the square cloth and tying the corners to make a handle.

futari two persons

futate two-handed

gammaku mid-section of the torso, obliques, and gluteal muscles

G

gasshuku training camp, group training event

gedan lower level

gedan barai downward block

geri see Keri

geri kata kicking technique/form

giri filial piety, a sense of duty or obligation arising from personal honor and pride

go hard, as in Go– Ju (In-Yo)

go no kokyu hard or forced breathing

gyaku opposite, reverse

gyaku tsuki a reverse strike

hachiji dachi stance with the feet in the shape of the character for eight, Hachi (八)

H

hai yes

haito uchi ridge-hand strike

hajime instruction to start, begin

hana nose

hane uke splitting block, from the verb "Haneru" to divide

hantai opposite

hara abdomen, belly

heiko parallel

heisoku dachi a stance with the feet, toes, and heels together

hidari left

higashi east

hiji elbow

hiji ate elbow strike

hikite the arm pulling back, going in the opposite direction as the technique. The retracting arm/hand.

hiku to pull

hikui low

hiza knee

hiza geri knee kick, striking with the knee

hogen dialect

hojo undo supplemental training

hombu dojo main branch, headquarters, dojo of a style or association

iki breath

I

in yo Ying Yang, inside outside

ippon ashi dachi single leg stance

ippon kumite a fight involving a single attack

irikumi inside fighting

Vocabulary

J

iro obi color belt
itten single point
jigotai fighting stance with the front foot forward and the rear foot at 45°
jiku ashi standing leg, supporting, or pivoting leg
jissen kumite a real attack
jiyu kumite free sparring
jodan age uke high block
jodan tsuki high punch
joseki senior section of the Dojo floor
ju soft, the counter to Go
juji uke "x" or cross block. In the shape of the character for ten, Ju (十)
junbi undo warm up exercises
jutsu art, often used in Kenjutsu or Karatejutsu to distinguish from Kendo and Karatedo

K

kakato heel
kakato geri heel kick
kake dachi hook stance
kakete a hooking hand technique
kaki jichi hook strike
kakidi see Kakete (Oki.)
kamae ready position, guard position
kamaete command given by an instructor to have the student to assume a guard position
kamiza the front of the dojo
kansetsu geri a kick striking a joint typically a knee
kansetsu waza joint locks
karatejutsu alternative reading for Todejutsu, often used to distinguish "old school" karate from more modern version.
kata form or shape
kata shoulder
kata pattern or mold
katai hard or stiff
katate single handed
keiko training, instruction
keikogi training uniform
keri kick, sometime pronounced Geri in compound words
keri waza kicking techniques
kibishi strict, severe
kihon basic, elementary, fundamental
kihon dosa fundamental movements
kihon kata basic form
kihon kumite basic two person practice
kihon waza basic technique
kime focus applied to a technique
kingeri groin kick
kinniku muscle
kintama testicles

ボキャブラリー　　　　　　　　　　　　　Vocabulary

kiotsuke command given by an instructor to have the students come to attention

kiru to cut

kohai junior

koi guchi carp's mouth. A term used in Kenjutsu for the shape of the hand when grabbing the scabbard. Used in Shinjinbukan to refer to the shape of the hand when grabbing an arm.

kokoro heart, spirit

kokustu dachi back-leaning stance

kokyu breathing technique

koshi waist, hips

koshi waza hip techniques

kote forearm

kotekitai forearm striking exercise

kubi neck

kukan tsuki air striking techniques

kukuchi muscular contraction with breathing technique

kukuma di circular hands (Oki.)

kumadi bear paw. A hand position in which the fingers and thumb are rolled halfway, creating a flat striking surface on the palm of the hand. (Oki.)

kumite sparring

kuro obi black belt

kuru in context of body mechanics often translated as "crank" when referring to the foot or leg

kushijikei hip rotation (Oki.)

kyukei a break, a pause

ma ushiro directly to the back

M

machi dojo a private Dojo

machiwara striking post, often pronounced in Japanese as Makiwara. Literally "wrapped straw" although post war Machiwara usually have leather rather than straw.

mae front, forward

mago deshi students who are second generation removed from a teacher, "grand student"

mannaka center, mid-point

matte command given by an instructor to have the student wait

mawashi circular, round

mawashi geri roundhouse kick

mawashi uke roundhouse block

mawatte to rotate, to spin

me eye(s)

mi jichi striking with the eyes, a technique for focusing when striking

michi way, path, road

miji nagashi jichi water flowing strike, a descending strike (Oki.)

mikazuki geri crescent kick

mimi ear

minami south

mizu nagashi tsuki Japanese pronunciation of "water flowing strike"

mokuso meditation

Vocabulary

morote two-handed, augmented hand technique

muchimi flexibility, suppleness as well as stickiness in executing a technique

mudansha a student who holds no Dan level rank

mune chest

mushin an empty or clear mind; a mind not fixed on anything and open to everything

musubi dachi open foot stance

N

naa garden used for training space, often in front of a teacher's home or family tomb

nafudakake name and rank board on the wall of a Dojo which indicates the hierarchy of ranks within that particular Dojo

nagashi jichi reaching strike

nagashi uke sweeping block

nakayubi middle finger

naore command given by an instructor to have the student "reset"

neko ashi dachi cat leg stance, cat stance

nidan geri two level kick, double jumping kick

ninen geiko (lit. two years' training) a tradition still held in many dojos. Practice is held from eleven in the evening until one in the morning on New Year's Eve.

nishi west

nobasu to reach out, lengthen, stretch, straighten

nodo throat

nukite spear hand

nuku to extract or remove

O

oi tsuki lunging strike

omote in the context of Shinjinbukan training, this refers to the "standard" direction of a Kata, as opposed to the reverse "Ura"

onegaishimasu (lit. if you please) It is often said before entering a dojo, as a way to ask for permission to enter, also when bowing to a training partner before practice begins.

osae uke pressing block

osaeru to hold down, restrict, control

otagai partner, peers

otagai ni rei bow to each other

otoshi uke a downward pushing block

oyayubi thumb

R

randori free flow exercise: training method used to learn to make techniques flow smoothly

reigi saho courtesy and manners / respect and etiquette

ren tsuki alternating punches

renoji dachi stance with the feet in the shape of the character "Re" (レ)

renshu to practice

renzoku geri continuous kicks

renzoku tsuki continuous striking (punches)

ritsu rei a semi-formal, standing shallow bow

rokusho six hands

ryou ashi both legs, both feet

ryou te two-handed

ryu style, (as in Shorin-ryu, Goju-ryu, Uechi-ryu)

ryu ha style and lineage. The style refers to the art while the lineage refers to the teacher.

ボキャブラリー — Vocabulary

S

sagi machiwara hanging Machiwara
sagurite no kamae searching hands ready position, also called bridging hand
saigo last
sakotsu collar bone, clavicle
sanchin dachi hour-glass stance
sankaku triangle
sankaku tenshin triangular walking pattern.
sawaru to touch
sayu right and left
sayu tsuki double side strike
seiken fist
seiken tsuki a straight strike
seiza kneeling position
sensei teacher or professor. Not an awarded title but a function or role.
senpai/sempai one's senior in rank or age
shibori squeezing technique
shiboru to squeeze
shidoin formal title for an accredited instructor
shihan a teacher of teachers, someone whose students are recognized instructors
shiko dachi wide stance with the feet out to 45°
shime originating from Shimeru (to close), the tension of muscles while executing a technique
shimeru to close, to tie
shimoseki lower part of a Dojo. The rear area where the junior students stand.
shinnen geiko New Year's training, the first practice of the new year
shita low, bottom
shita tongue
shita tsuki a low strike, a strike to the lower abdomen
shizen natural, nature
shizen dachi natural position
shizuka quiet
shoga ken ginger fist
shomen the front wall of the school, the place of honor in a Dojo. Usually where a shrine, scroll, or picture is hung.
shomen ni rei instruction to bow towards the front
shotei ate palm-heel smash
shugyo ascetic exercise
shukyo religion
shuto uchi knife-hand or sword-hand strike
shuto uke knife-hand block
shuugou to come together, to assemble, command given by an instructor to have the student line-up
soji cleaning
soko ashi the arch of the foot
sokuto the edge of the foot
sokutsu dachi outside leaning stance
soto gedan barai outside downward block

Vocabulary

soto ude uke outside forearm block
soto uke outward mid-section block
suihei flat, horizontal, level
sureru to rub, to graze
suri ashi sliding footwork
suwaru to sit
tachi See Dachi
tachi machiwara standing Machiwara
taketaba a training tool consisting of a bundle of thin bamboo
tanden also called Hara, point about 2cm below the navel
tate hiza a position in which one knee is on the floor, while the other leg has the foot flat on the floor and the knee up
tate tsuki a vertical strike, where vertical refers to the position of the fist
tate uke a vertical block where vertical refers to the position of the forearm
tatsu to stand, to get on one's feet
tazuna no kamae "bridle" Kamae
te hand
te (Ty, Ti) generic term for Okinawan fighting arts
te waza hand technique
tettsui hammer fist; a strike with the pinky finger side of a closed fist
tettsui uchi bottom of the fist, or hammer fist strike
ti hand (Oki.)
ti machiwara handheld machiwara
tijigaya a person who is capable of using Ti (Oki.)
tijikun a fist strike (Oki.)
tobi (Tobu) jump
tode China hand, also pronounces Toudi
togu to sharpen, used to mean perfect a technique
tomeru to stop
tora guchi tiger's mouth
tori the person countering the attack in partner training
tsuki strike
tsuki kata punching form or technique
tsuki waza punching technique
tsumasaki tips of the toes
tsuru ashi dachi crane stance
tsuyoi strong
uchi interior, inner
uchi barai inside sweeping block
uchi deshi live-in disciple, closed-door student
uchi otoshi striking block
uchi uke inward mid-section block
uchi uke otoshi inward mid-section pushing block
uchinanchu an Okinawan person (Oki.)

Vocabulary

uchinanguchi the Okinawan language (Oki.)
ude arm
udi arm (Oki.)
ue up, upper, above
uke block
uke ashi dachi blocking stance
uke kata blocking form/technique
ukutsu dachi inside leaning stance
ura reverse side
uraken backfist
urati back of the fist, also pronounced Uradi (Oki.)
uratijikun a backfist strike (Oki.)
ushiro back
utsu to hit someone
wakeru to divide, to separate
waki armpit
waza technique
yakusoku pre-arranged
yama no gamae upper-level guard with arms apart in the shape of the kanji for mountain, Yama (山)
yama tsuki strike in the shape of the kanji character for mountain, Yama (山)
yame command given by an instructor to have the student stop
yasumu to rest
yawarakai soft
yo outside, as in in-yo
yoi ready position
yoko side
yoko geri side kick
yoko geri keage side snap kick
yoko geri kekomi side thrust kick
yoko tobi geri jumping side kick
yori ashi shuffling, advancing without changing the relative position of the feet
yubi finger
zanshin mental alertness
zarei kneeling bow from seiza
zazen sitting meditation
zenkutsu dachi forward leaning stance

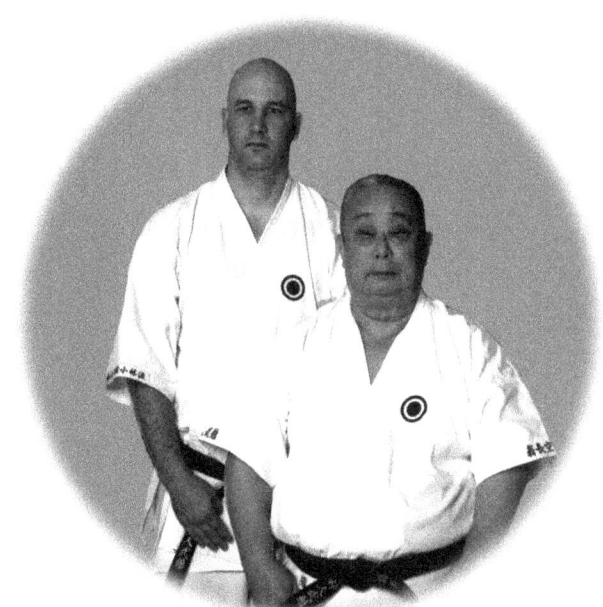

Daniel Kogan, chief instructor of the Pine Lake branch of the Shinjinbukan Karate Dojo, with Yoshimitsu Onaga, the founder and head instructor of the Shinjinbukan Shorin-ryu Dojo in Naha, Okinawa, Japan.

(Photo taken in Issaquah, Washington, USA, in 2009 during the photoshoot for the Japanese language publication 神人武館教書 *Shinjinbukan Textbook vol 1,2,3*)

www.ingramcontent.com/pod-product-compliance
Lightning Source LLC
Chambersburg PA
CBHW041244240426
43670CB00027B/2986